The Weight-Loss Book for People Who Hate Exercise

EXERCISE SUCKS!

The Secret to
Losing Weight
Without
Really Trying

From Wellness Expert & Celebrity Trainer

KENT BURDEN

Exercise Sucks!

Exercise Sucks!

The Secret to Losing Weight without Really Trying

By Kent Burden

Editor: Jessica Sarra

Published 2012 by MLF Press, a subsidiary of My Life Fitness, LLC

ISBN#: 978-1480206175

Table of Contents

Our Free Gift to You!

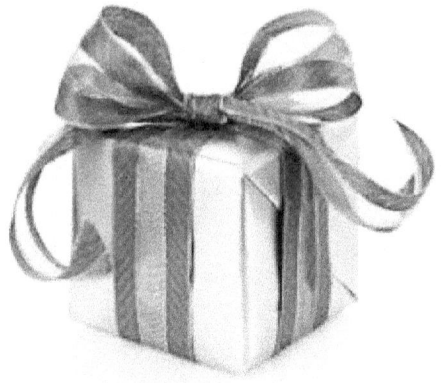

7 Days of Delicious Real Food Dinner Recipes

www.mylifefitness.com/7realfooddinners

Introduction

Exercise Sucks!

Let's face it, for most people the title of this book pretty much sums up how they feel about exercise: *Exercise Sucks!* And what's not to hate? There's all the sweating, grunting, discomfort and the workout wear that shows off all the ripples and bulges we try so hard to conceal. And going to the gym is pure, unadulterated hell! It smells like rubber and sweat, there are all the machines you have absolutely no idea how to use, and some freak is bellowing at the top of his lungs as he tries to press an ungodly amount of weight off his chest. Over in the corner some chick in a sports bra and bike shorts is hitting on one of the trainers and you feel like everyone is staring at you. No, for most of us exercise is no picnic.

The problem is that without some sort of daily activity, something to get our heart pumping and our muscles activated we tend to go a little…well, soft. Our backsides begin to grow wide, threatening to need their own area codes. Our bellies begin to expand so we can't see our shoes. Quite frankly nobody wants that, especially not you. The trick is figuring out how to avoid *both* of these unappealing scenarios. How do you keep your body fit while at the same avoiding the gym or exhausting workouts? Well, if you want to lose some weight while doing the minimum amount of grueling, high-intensity, kick-your-booty working out, you've bought the right book!

It's not that you won't have to do a little exercise; after all, for the last 20 years my job as a certified master wellness coach and celebrity trainer has been to torture people (including Drew Barrymore, Julia Roberts, Alanis Morissette, and Clint Black) into looking hot and sexy for the camera. I would be derelict in my duties (and drummed out of the personal trainer secret fraternity) if I didn't give you a little love, too. But this book is based on the new science of "sedentary studies" and a new disorder that doctors call "sitting disease." I have to tell you that the findings of this new research have really knocked me for a loop.

I spent a great deal of my professional life playing by the rules: 30-45 minutes of sustained cardio, a healthy dose of strength training, toss in some flexibility exercises, then forget about it and go about your day.

Most of my clients worked hard and got great results, but occasionally I did have a *problem* client. Not that they didn't work hard, but perhaps they had trouble losing that last 10 or 15 pounds or they just couldn't get their blood work numbers under control. All of my training told me I was doing the right things but nothing seemed to work. This was really troubling for me (I mean, I was charging a LOT of money for these sessions so I wanted people to be successful and happy) and I found myself trying new exercises and different training techniques, but to no avail. I tried to shrug it off and tell myself they weren't following their nutrition program or they were cheating and not doing their cardio on days that we didn't work together. But they said they *were* doing those things and deep down inside I didn't think they were lying to me. Then one day in 2010 I had an "aha!" moment.

While reading a popular men's magazine I stumbled across an article on "sitting disease." The article talked about a growing body of research that pointed to sitting as an independent risk factor for metabolic diseases and weight gain regardless of the amount of exercise an individual did. So I went back in my records and, lo and behold, all of my "problem" clients had jobs that had them sitting for most of the day. There was the financial planner, the mortgage broker, the lawyer, and the computer programmer. While all of these people were working out for 60 minutes every day, they would also spend 7 to 11 hours a day sitting in front of a computer at work and then another hour or two (or three or four) relaxing on the couch as they watched a little television after work. It was after this realization that I decided to find out as much as I could about this "sitting disease."

The information I discovered is what makes this book so much different from other exercise and weight loss books on the market today. This book takes a completely different approach to helping you shed those unwanted pounds and helping you look and feel better than you ever have before. Rather than focusing on the small percentage of your day where you "work out," we are going to focus on getting you more active over the course of the entire day. We will also take a look at your eating habits, give you insights on how to eat healthier with real food that tastes good (no weird diets or shakes here), and even throw in some tips on foods that will rev up your metabolism and actually help you lose weight.

I want to be honest with you: If you want a body that looks like Dara Torres or Ryan Reynolds (you know what I mean: ripped, tight, and toned with washboard abs), you are going to have to do some serious dieting and spend a lot of time in the gym, because that is how you get a body that looks like that. But if you just want to lose that spare tire, whittle off some of the jiggle from your rear end, or drop several pant or dress sizes, then this is the weight loss program for you.

I've tried to keep this book short and to the point because I know we're all very busy people and we don't have a lot of time to read through tons of research and study endless streams of data. You want to know what to do and why you should do it; Plain and simple. So let's get started!

Exercise Sucks!

Chapter 1
What the Science has to Say

Most people think that to lose weight they have to turn their lives upside down and empty their wallets. There's joining the gym, hiring a personal trainer, and making room in your hectic schedule to fit that hour of exercise in. Then of course there is the thought of the exercise itself. An hour of physical and emotional torture with a dash of humiliation as you are forced to do things you neither like nor are particularly good at. Let's not forget that you will also need to change the way you eat. You can eat like a Neanderthal, go raw vegan, or maybe just choke down one of those chalky gritty shakes a couple of times a day. Oh yeah, for some of us the thought of trying to lose weight ranks right up there with going to the dentist for a root canal or, even worse, spending two weeks in a deserted mountain cabin with the in-laws.

But what if I told you it didn't have to be like that? What if you could lose weight just by adding some simple movements to your day that can be done almost anywhere, take no more than 5 minutes an hour to do, and don't even require that you break a sweat. Then you're free to just do the things you already do every day, but do them in a slightly different way. Add to that the fact that you could eat really yummy food that tastes great and you would never feel deprived.

Sound too good to be true? Well it's not. And no, this isn't some crazy idea I came up with after bursting a blood vessel in my brain while trying to bench press way too much weight. This program is based on real science from some of the most prestigious universities in the world such as the Mayo clinic, the Pennington Biomedical Research Center, University College London, University of Sydney, and the University of Missouri.

The pioneer in this research is Dr. James Levine of the Mayo clinic who has devoted twenty plus years of his life to the study of NEAT. NEAT, or *non-exercise activity thermogenesis,* is a really fancy way of describing the movements that make up your daily life. Not exercise, but stuff like walking to the bathroom, picking up the stapler, standing up when your boss comes into your cubicle, running the vacuum in the living room, chewing gum, and even picking your nose. It is these everyday movements, not exercise, which made our forefathers "active."

In fact, historically speaking, exercise as we know it was an anomaly, not the norm.

What Dr. Levine has discovered in those twenty plus years is that we are doing less NEAT movements and a lot more sitting. The problem is that sitting is one of the most sedentary things you can do and as a society, we do more sitting today than ever before in human history. It hardly seems a coincidence that we are also heavier today than at any other time in human history.

For decades scientists have studied the relationship between how much we exercise, how often we exercise and our health. In the last five years, however, some scientists have begun looking at this correlation from a different perspective: Instead of thinking about what *exercise* does *for* the body, researches started to investigate what *sitting* for long periods of time does *to* the body. This was some seriously unconventional thinking.

Rather than looking at what we *weren't* doing, they started to look at what we *were* doing, which was a heck of a lot of sitting. In fact, by some estimates many people are sitting as much as 12 hours a day. This new perspective has begun to turn the science of sedentary studies on its head. Researchers from such diverse fields as epidemiology, molecular biology, biomechanics, and physiology are seeing data that is leading them to believe that the amount of sitting we do on a daily basis may not only be making us very fat, it could also be causing us to die prematurely. The most disturbing revelation is that 30-60 minutes of sustained exercise a day may have little or no positive affect on a sedentary lifestyle. To put it simply, sitting for extended periods of time may be slowly killing you, and just working out after sitting around all day may not be enough to save you.

The fact that sitting around is bad for you isn't very surprising; you would have to be living under a rock not to have heard that doing nothing for long periods of time could make you fat and unhealthy. Most of us think that if we hop on a treadmill, take a spin class, or shake our groove thing in a Zumba class a few times a week, we're in the clear. But according to microbiologist Marc T. Hamilton, PhD from the University of Missouri, we need to adjust our thought process. "People need to understand that the qualitative mechanisms of sitting are completely different from walking or exercising...Sitting too much is not the same as exercising too little. They do completely different things to the body."

In a 2005 article in *Science* magazine, Dr. Levine gave his insights into why, despite similar diets, some people are fat and others aren't. "We found that people with obesity have a natural predisposition to be attracted to the chair, and that's true even after obese people lose weight," he says. "What fascinates me is that humans evolved over 1.5 million years entirely on the ability to walk and move. And literally 150 years ago, 90% of human endeavor was still agricultural. In a tiny speck of time we've become "chair-sentenced," Levine says. This "chair sentence" may very well be a death sentence.

So what's the big difference between sitting and standing, you ask? I mean just standing around seems every bit as lazy as sitting, doesn't it? Dr. Hamilton knows better. "If you're standing around and puttering, you recruit specialized muscles designed for postural support that never tire," he says. "They're unique in that the nervous system recruits them for low-intensity activity and they're very rich in enzymes." One such enzyme, lipoprotein lipase, sucks fat and cholesterol from the blood stream, and burns the fat for energy while shifting the cholesterol from LDL (the bad kind of cholesterol) to HDL (the healthy kind of cholesterol). When you're sitting, the muscles are relaxed, and enzyme activity drops by 90 to 95%, leaving fat to hang out in the bloodstream. After a couple hours of sitting, healthy cholesterol drops by 20%. Amazingly this is just one of the myriad chemical changes that take place in the body while we sit. Sitting for extended periods of time has a huge cascade of effects on the body, everything from back pain and restricted blood flow to being implicated in an elevated risk of certain kinds of cancer.

As fascinating as I find the biochemistry and health implications of a sedentary lifestyle, the focus of this book is weight loss (but if you're as big a geek as I am, and want to find out more about the damage sitting does to your overall health, you can read my book *Is Your Chair Killing You?* available on Amazon at: tinyurl.com/9r74tgp

The reason you probably bought this book is that you or someone you care about needs to lose a few pounds...maybe more than a few. Well, you're not alone. Today more than two- thirds of Americans are overweight and roughly one-third of us are obese. But it hasn't always been this way. In fact, just 50 years ago the average American weighed 26 pounds less than today. Another thing that has changed drastically in the last 50 years is the way most of us work. According to the Centers for Disease Control and Prevention's weekly *Morbidity and Mortality Report*, most Americans get very little or no physical activity during the work day, and in fact only 6.5% of all U.S. adults meet the "minimum activity guidelines" while at work.

A study published in May 2011 by peer-reviewed science journal PLos ONE shows that since 1960 jobs that require physical movement have slowly disappeared. Today, less than 20% of private sector jobs require "moderate" activity; that's a whopping 30% less than in the early 1960s. To underscore how sedentary we've become, look at the 2008 study by researchers at the National Institute of Health who had 6,000 American adults strap on accelerometers to see just how much they moved over the course of the day (*moved,* not exercised). They determined that less than 5% got in 30 minutes of continuous physical activity five days a week. Equally disturbing is the study published in the *American Journal of Epidemiology* in 2008. This study, which followed 6,329 people, found that 60% of our waking hours are spent in sedentary pursuits like sitting at a desk or driving to work. The bottom line is: we're strapped to our chairs and it's making our fannies fat and our bellies bulge.

Work is not the only thing that's keeping our bottoms firmly rooted in the seated position. Let's take a look at what the statistics say about how we spend our time at home, starting with television. According to the Nielsen Company, the average American watches more than four hours of TV each day—that's 28 hours per week, or two months of TV watching per year! In a 65-year lifespan, an average American will have spent nine years glued to the television. *Nine years*…these days, most marriages don't last that long!

According to an eye-opening new analysis done by researchers at the University of California, Berkeley, Americans spend nine times as many minutes watching TV or movies as they do participating in sports, exercise and all other leisure-time physical activities combined. When looking at which activities contributed more to energy expenditure among Americans, the researchers found that driving a car, watching TV, and working in an office outranked sports and heart-pumping workouts. In this study, which was released by the *International Journal of Behavioral Nutrition,* lead author Linda Dong notes that

[t]his study provides a wake-up call for the nation, particularly in light of rising obesity rates in this country. A lot of people aren't fully aware of how sedentary their lives are. This paper shows that, as a population, leisure-time physical activities are at the bottom of our priority lists.

The study appears to provide the first national scale, quantitative analysis of energy expenditure in the United States. The paper comes during an epidemic of obesity in this country, and at a time when federal health officials are reporting that poor diet and physical inactivity are quickly gaining on smoking as leading causes of preventable deaths.

So how did the researchers come to find all of this data? The UC Berkeley researchers used data from 7,515 adults questioned from 1992 to 1994 for the National Human Activity Pattern Survey (NHAPS). Those surveyed were asked to report everything they did and how long they did it during the prior 24 hours. More than 125,500 reports of activities were grouped into 255 categories that were similar in the energy required to do them. The researchers collected information on how many people reported doing each activity, how long they did it, and how much energy it took to do it. From this information, it was possible to estimate total energy expended on each activity. The study found that, outside of sleeping, the largest collective contributor to energy expenditure among the population was driving a car, followed by office work, and watching TV, partly because so many people reported those activities. In contrast, leisure-time physical activity, such as jogging or playing basketball, accounted for only 5% of the population's total energy expenditure. It doesn't take a rocket scientist, or a Berkeley researcher for that matter, to figure out that cutting back on the time spent watching TV or movies would free up precious minutes for exercise.

But it's not just the television gobbling up our downtime and keeping our butts glued to the couch after we get home from work; social networking sites are fast becoming a popular attraction as well. According to The Nielsen Company, individual global consumers spent an average of more than five and a half hours on social networking sites like Facebook and Twitter in December 2009. This represents an 82% increase from the same time in December 2008, when users were spending just over three hours on social networking sites. Globally, social networks and blogs are the most popular online category when ranked by average time spent in

December, followed by online games and instant messaging. With 206.9 million unique visitors, Facebook was the number one global social networking destination in December 2009, and 67% of global social media users visited the site at least once during the month. The amount of time spent on Facebook continues to rise, with global users spending nearly six hours per month on the site. In the U.S., it's not just young Americans using these social networking sites; geezers are now getting seriously into the act as well. According to Nielson, Americans over the age of 50 visited social networking sites twice as often as kids under 18!

So let's see if we can break down all this statistical mumbo jumbo: For the most part, it looks like the majority of us spend more time than ever in a seated position, sitting at our desks hunched over a computer screen, only getting up to use the bathroom and eat. Then most of us head home and watch some television or visit social networking sites like Facebook, My Space, LinkedIn or Twitter, and we do it all while firmly planted in the seated position.

I know, I know, I said I wasn't going to give you a whole bunch of research and data. But I think it's really important to understand just how sedentary we've become, because this is the key to how we are going to lose those unwanted pounds without going to the gym or spending a ton of time "exercising."

Now that we know what the problem is, it's time to talk about solutions. This is where things get interesting, because this is where we bridge the gap between past failures and future success. This is where we replace an old model that doesn't work with a new model that taps into the way our bodies were designed to function and gets you the results you've always dreamed of. This isn't a miracle cure, it will take time and discipline. But if you stick with it you will lose the weight, feel more energetic, and be healthier than you have ever been before.

Chapter 2

Real Food

How to Eat to Lose Weight and be Healthier

If you think *Exercise Sucks* then nutrition becomes a critical factor to the success of losing weight. There's an old saying among trainers: "you can't exercise your way out of a bad diet," and it's true. But with all the fad diets out there, and all the so called experts touting their weight loss plans, and all the "health food gurus" and infomercial darlings filling the air waves, how do you know what nutritional program is right for you? I don't know. Not really what you wanted to hear, right? But it's the truth: I don't know.

But let's talk about what I *do* know. I know that I am not a nutritionist, nor am I a registered dietitian. I am, however, a guy who has been fascinated by nutrition his whole life (I'm one of those geeks who actually reads diet and nutrition books on the beach for fun) and I'm actually half way through the curriculum for my master's degree in nutrition.

To date most of my research in nutrition has left me feeling like Albert Einstein must have felt when he said "the more I learn the less I know." And that, my friends, is the LAST time I will ever compare myself to Albert Einstein. The topic of nutrition can seem so simple (calories in, calories out) yet so complex (how the body extracts nutrients and energy from food). Now toss in personal body chemistry (food allergies and sensitivities) and personal taste (you hate vegetables) and you can see why there are literally thousands of different nutritional theories.

And most importantly, who's to say which one is right for you?

Well, I actually have the answer for that last question. Who's to say which one is right for you? You are! Whether it be Paleo, vegetarian, Mediterranean, Okinawa, vegan, raw or whatever, with a little experimentation and a lot of listening to your body you can decide what kind of eating program fits your lifestyle, tastes, and weight loss goals. If one program leaves you listless and constantly hungry try another. If you simply can't eat another salad, move on. Can't afford endless plates of steaks and bacon…you get the idea. Figuring out what works for you can be fun, exciting, and downright tasty.

Having said all that, there really isn't any reason you have to choose any eating program, diet, or fad. You could just follow some basic principles that can lead you in the direction of eating the kinds of foods that will be good for you and help you lose weight in such a way that you can keep it off.

1. Eat real food

What's real food, you say? Real food is something your great, great, great grandmother would have cooked for her family. It's made from real ingredients and it's fresh. It's not industrialized food. It doesn't have a bunch of ingredients listed on the box that you can't pronounce and it wasn't made in a factory. The best food is usually pretty simple and it tastes great. Stuff like fresh fruit, fresh or frozen vegetables, whole grains, lean meats and fish, olive oil and butter. These are all real foods. Why is this important? Well, as a society we started gaining weight just about the time we started to industrialize our food supply…coincidence? I don't believe in coincidence. Pre-packaged food tends to be loaded with fat, sugar, and salt, not to mention fillers, artificial colors, and preservatives. How does the combination of these ingredients affect our bodies? Nobody is really certain but we do know one thing: They aren't making us skinny, which is what most of our ancestors who ate real food were. For more information about real food and its benefits, I recommend checking out the book *Real Food* by Nina Planck.

2. Eat lots of nutrient-dense, naturally low-calorie foods

Foods that are loaded with vitamins, minerals, antioxidants, and fiber, but are low in calories, would seem to be super-duper diet foods, wouldn't you think? Fresh fruits and vegetables fit this description to a tee. They fill you up, taste great, and energize and power you up for the day, yet they are low in calories, amazing!

3. Get enough protein and fat

Protein helps build muscle and helps to keep us feeling full. Fat is crucial (especially essential fatty acids) to many of our bodily functions and makes us feel satisfied after eating it. These key nutritional elements don't have to come from animal products (if you are vegetarian or vegan you can get protein from tofu or rice and beans, and essential fatty acids from nuts, seeds, and certain plants like flax or purslane) but must be a part of a healthy diet.

4. Don't stuff yourself

Eat until you are 80% full. You should never leave the table feeling like Fat Bastard in the *Austin Powers* movie. Just about the time you start to feel satisfied, stop eating. Just because it's on your plate doesn't mean you have to eat it. That is especially true at restaurants, where portion sizes can be extremely large. I'm not going to get into the whole psychology of why you may have been programmed to "clean your plate," but if that is a problem for you, then work on it.

5. Don't just shovel it in

Take your time and enjoy your food. Slowing yourself down during a meal accomplishes two things. One, you'll do a better job of chewing your food and thus aid digestion. Two, it takes about twenty minutes for your stomach to get the signal to your brain that you're full, so by slowing down the eating process, you are less likely to overindulge.

6. Live by the 70/30 rule

The 70/30 rule is 70% of what you eat comes from plant-based sources (mostly fresh fruit and vegetables with a sprinkling of whole grains) and 30% from animal sources (eggs, fish, lean meats, and dairy). It is believed by many anthropologists that this was the ratio of food intake for our early ancestors.

7. Become an avid reader

Of food labels that is. Reading labels can be a real eye opener. Not only should you know what the calorie count is for your meal, but you should also know what the ingredients are. If you can't pronounce it you probably shouldn't be eating it. Knowledge is power and that statement is especially true when it comes to eating for weight loss.

8. Get a handle on portion size

Learning to eyeball your portion sizes can be incredibly helpful in curbing overeating. A great way to start getting a feel for portion size is to close your eyes and visualize holding a baseball in your hand. (Not into the whole woojie visualization thing? Grab an actual baseball.) Now open your eyes and grab a handful of broccoli. The amount of broccoli in your hand should roughly be about the same size as the baseball. Now put that handful of broccoli on a plate and really take a minute or two to see how much room that broccoli takes up on the plate. That, my friends, is a serving. Now try putting a stacked deck of cards on a plate. Become aware of just how much space that deck takes up. A deck of cards is about the size of a 3-4 ounce portion of meat, which is one serving. Web MD has a great portion slide show on its website at the following link:

http://www.webmd.com/diet/healthtool-portion-size-plate

9. Be Colorful

No, I don't mean be eccentric like my Uncle Frank. I mean fill your plate with color. The colors in our food actually indicate what type and how much of specific antioxidants and phytonutrients the food contains. Colors like red, orange, purple, yellow, blue, and deep greens should be a large part of your diet every day.

10. Dump the refined sugar, high-fructose corn syrup, and white flour

I know. This is the toughest one for most people because they seem to be in everything you buy that comes in a package. But these three things are probably the biggest contributors to weight gain and the inability to shed unwanted pounds. I refer you back to #1 on this list. Your great, great, great grandmother probably used honey or unrefined sugar as well as whole wheat flour, and probably even used these ingredients sparingly because they were expensive.

11. Avoid fast food like the plague

If you're trying to lose weight your local drive through is the devil. I know--I often hear the siren song of my local burger joint as I drive by on my way home from work. The food tastes good and sometimes I really don't feel like cooking. But one look at the calorie count on your favorite combo meal should send you screaming into the night. It's important to remember the weight gain factor from fast foods extends beyond the calorie count. These foods tend to be made with highly processed ingredients like white flour, preservatives, chemical fillers, sodium, colors and tons of refined sugar and high-fructose corn syrup. If you take a look at #10 you'll see why you should stay away from fast food.

12. Think before you drink

Beverages can be the stealth bomber that flies in under the radar and destroys your weight loss efforts. When trying to lose weight, be *VERY* mindful of what you drink. A 12oz can of soda has between 140-165 calories and is loaded with high fructose corn syrup. A large coke (32oz) at your local fast food establishment has 310 calories. And substituting a diet soda for a regular one may not be a great solution.

According to an article by Dr. Oz, "Most diet sodas are lower in calories than regular soda because they don't use regular sugar. The problem here is the artificial sweeteners, which have been tied to weight gain. Why?

Research shows that artificial sweeteners stimulate taste receptors that sense sweetness in both the esophagus and stomach. Anticipating energy, the pancreas releases insulin, an important hormone for accumulating body fat. At the same time, chemicals are sent to the brain's satiety center, which becomes confused as to whether or not the body is actually receiving calories.

As your body gets "tricked" by the sugar substitute, you crave more food and become susceptible to overeating in order to feel satisfied. The result? You feel even hungrier and less full, which can lead to weight gain."

Now I'm going to say right up front that the studies that he is basing this on are small and not yet fully accepted but you've already learned that artificial ingredients aren't a healthy thing for your body and that there are far better choices than diet soda.

Sodas aren't the only sneaky beverage that can tempt you into sabotaging your weight loss. Did you know that a Grande Blended Mocha Frappucchino with whipped cream has a whopping 420 calories? Alcoholic beverages are high in calories as well.

I suggest water, tea and coffee as great weight loss beverages (in the next section you'll see why). Not a big fan of water? Try a refreshing spritzer made of sparkling water jazzed up with a squeeze of lemon, lime or just a splash of fruit juice (my favorites are tart cherry, cranberry and pomegranate). The bottom line is that whatever you decide to drink, think about whether it's helping your weight loss efforts or hindering them. Then sit back enjoy it.

Real Food Weight Loss Helpers

Keep in mind that food can be more than just sustenance. As Hippocrates said "Let food be thy medicine and medicine be thy food." The following list of foods can actually double as weight-loss drugs (without the nasty side effects), helping to boost your metabolism and speed up your weight loss. Even better, they're good for you and taste great!

Green tea

In a study by the American Journal of Physiology, Regulatory, Integrative and Comparative Physiology found that drinking green tea was believed to keep the metabolism from slowing which often accompanies weight loss. The authors of this same report found that green tea seems to have the ability to inhibit the effects of catechol-o-methyltransferase which is an enzyme known to start the process of breaking down certain brain chemicals involved in the regulation of the appetite.

Another study published in 2009 in the International Journal of Obesity found that some antioxidants in green tea appear to have a "small positive effect" on both weight loss and weight maintenance. Their analysis of 11 studies on green tea found that green tea antioxidants known as catechins seemed to help increase metabolism.

Cinnamon

It appears that cinnamon has a regulatory effect on blood sugar levels as well as raising insulin levels in the body. It is believed to do this by imitating the biological activity of insulin as well as increasing the metabolism of glucose. It's been proven that high blood sugar levels can lead to the storage of fat which means that cinnamon may help decrease the storing of fat, thus helping you lose weight. Cinnamon helps to slow the passing of food from the stomach to the intestines, keeping you feeling full longer. Cinnamon can help the body process carbohydrates more efficiently which of course may help you shed a few pounds, especially around the middle since abdominal fat is more sensitive to the effects of cinnamon than fat from around other areas of the body.

Peppers

Peppers (both the hot and the sweet varieties) have been shown to increase the body's heat production as well as oxygen consumption for as much as 20 minutes after they are consumed. This means your body is burning extra calories, which helps with weight loss. Granted the calorie burn isn't huge but every little bit helps.

Coffee

While the caffeine in coffee gives your metabolism a boost coffee's weight loss effect goes beyond just caffeine. Coffee, which happens to be one of the most widely consumed beverages in the world, contains a ton of naturally-occurring compounds, including several classes of antioxidants. Coffee is already known to be a preventive factor against mild depression, Parkinson's disease, and colon and rectal cancers. Now it looks as though the compounds in coffee also help to regulate blood glucose, reduce fat production, and enable steady weight loss.

Grapefruit

Remember the Grapefruit Diet? According to an article on About.com, written by Mary Shannon, they may have been on to something. The article states: "With its high fiber content and low glycemic load, grapefruit may be a secret weight-loss weapon. Research suggests that dieters might be more successful if they select foods with staying power like whole citrus that help curb appetite and prevent overeating. That's what a new study by the Nutrition and Metabolic Research Center at Scripps Clinic has confirmed. Researchers there found that the simple act of adding grapefruit and grapefruit juice to one's diet can result in weight loss.

The 12-week pilot study, led by Dr. Ken Fujioka, monitored weight and metabolic factors, such as insulin secretion, of the 100 men and women who participated in the Scripps Clinic 'Grapefruit Diet' study. On average, participants who ate half a grapefruit with each meal lost 3.6 pounds, while those who drank a serving of grapefruit juice three times a day lost 3.3 pounds. However, many patients in the study lost more than 10 pounds.

Additionally, the research indicates a physiological link between grapefruit and insulin, as it relates to weight management. The researchers speculate that the chemical properties of grapefruit reduce insulin levels and encourage weight loss. The importance of this link lies with the hormone's weight management function. While not its primary function, insulin assists with the regulation of fat metabolism. Therefore, the smaller the insulin spike after a meal, the more efficiently the body processes food for use as energy and the less it's stored as fat in the body. Grapefruit may possess unique chemical properties that reduce insulin levels which promotes weight loss." -About.com.

Oatmeal

Were you aware that by simply eating breakfast you increase your metabolism by 10%? Make your breakfast a bowl of oatmeal and that percentage goes up even higher. Because it takes a long time to break down all the water soluble fiber in oatmeal your body uses more energy getting the job done. This also means that you feel fuller longer, helping you avoid that mid-morning snack.

Curry

The ingredient in curry that gives it that distinctive bright yellow color is turmeric, and turmeric is loaded with curcumin. A study recently published in the Journal of Nutrition by Asma Ejaz and colleagues from Tufts University, Boston, MA, suggests that curcumin may also reduce fat formation by blocking the angiogenesis (growth of new blood vessels) necessary for the expansion of fat tissue and by positively changing fat cell metabolism. The researchers studied the effect of curcumin on mice that were fed a high-fat diet. Over 12 weeks, curcumin did not affect food intake but reduced body weight gain, adiposity, and micro-vessel density in the fat tissue of these mice. Curcumin treatment also increased expression of key enzymes involved in fat oxidation and lowered blood cholesterol levels.

The authors speculate that in humans, dietary curcumin may not only help prevent obesity, but may also have favorable effects on fat metabolism. What exactly does all that mean? Eating some good Indian food on a regular basis may be a great way to get and keep a flat belly.

Apples

In the old days they used to say "An apple a day keeps the doctor away." But today it actually looks like it may help keep the fat away as well. Apples are low in calories, fat, sodium and fiber, but high in nutrients. They help keep you feeling full while also keeping you from holding onto water weight. The vitamins and minerals will help keep your energy up and make you feel vibrant and ready to move.

Beans

Beans, beans, they're good for your heart. The more you eat, the more...the more weight you lose, apparently! The bottom line is that beans are high in protein, high in fiber and low in fat which keeps you feeling full and satisfied for a long time. Eating beans on a regular basis is a great strategy for weight loss because it may keep you from snacking. So eating beans at every meal may just be a great weight loss strategy—if your significant other can take the smell.

When you're trying to lose weight it can sometimes start to feel like food is your enemy. But the truth is, food is really your friend. Just like a good friend it can give you great pleasure, it can sustain you, and it can keep you healthy. It's important, though, to keep your relationship with your friend food balanced. You can't expect it to ease your pain or drown your sorrows. Your friend is not your crutch; it's your partner in good health.

To get you started on a new, healthy relationship with food, I have created a one week sample menu for you. This menu was meant to give you ideas on what kinds of food choices are available to you. It does not take into consideration food allergies or individual preferences, but will help you see how you can eat in a healthy and enjoyable way that can also help you lose weight.

So, since we all know that only a dietician or a nutritionist can prescribe a menu for health and weight loss, the following menu is for educational purposes only. Actually, it's just for fun.

Day 1

Breakfast: Steel cut oats with cinnamon and brown sugar, one half grapefruit, 1 mug of green tea

Optional Morning Snack: ¼ cup walnuts or almonds, 1 mug of green tea

Lunch: Whole grain pita turkey Mediterranean sandwich (pita, Greek yogurt, turkey, cucumber, red onion, tomato, spinach, olives), hummus and celery sticks

Optional Afternoon Snack: Cottage cheese with diced tomatoes

Dinner: Salad (spinach and tomato) with balsamic vinaigrette dressing, 4 ounce pork chop, sweet potato, peas

Dessert: Sorbet

Day 2

Breakfast: 2 boiled eggs, whole wheat toast, 1 cup bananas, 1 mug of green tea

Optional Morning Snack: Hummus & carrot sticks, 1 mug of green tea

Lunch: Tuna salad with whole wheat pasta (tuna, yogurt, celery, onion, lemon juice and whole wheat macaroni on a bed of arugula with balsamic vinaigrette)

Optional Afternoon Snack: ¼ cup almonds, 1 mug of green tea

Dinner: Salad (romaine lettuce, green pepper, onion, and balsamic vinaigrette), pot roast with onions, potatoes, and carrots.

Dessert: Baked apples

Day 3

Breakfast: Whole wheat bagel and lox with tomato, onion, spinach, 1 mug of green tea

Optional Morning Snack: Baked potato chips

Lunch: 1 cup chicken chili, mixed green salad with balsamic vinaigrette

Snack: Edamame

Dinner: Salad of sliced tomato and cucumber, chicken curry, spinach, brown rice

Dessert: Sliced apples with goat cheese

Day 4

Breakfast: Steel cut oats with blueberries, brown sugar, and cinnamon, 1 cup of coffee

Optional Morning Snack: Greek yogurt with strawberries

Lunch: Half a grapefruit, tomato and avocado salad, grilled cheese sandwich on whole wheat bread

Optional Afternoon Snack: Deviled eggs

Dinner: Mango, jicama, and cucumber salad, grilled shrimp tacos

Dessert: Chocolate tapioca pudding

Day 5

Breakfast: 2 poached eggs, half a grapefruit, whole wheat toast, 1 cup of coffee

Optional Morning Snack: Sliced pear with string cheese, 1 mug of green tea

Lunch: Black bean soup, corn and flaxseed tortilla chips

Optional Afternoon Snack: Roasted pumpkin seeds, grapefruit juice

Dinner: Caprese salad, whole wheat spaghetti with spinach marinara sauce

Dessert: Decaf espresso with grated dark chocolate

Day 6

Breakfast: Whole wheat breakfast cereal with milk, half a grapefruit, 1 cup of coffee

Optional Morning Snack: Veggie sushi roll

Lunch: Tomato soup, ham sandwich on whole wheat bread

Optional Afternoon Snack: Pretzels with honey mustard, 1 mug of green tea

Dinner: Arugula salad with sliced pears and goat cheese, grilled salmon, quinoa, sautéed Brussels sprouts

Dessert: Fruit plate

Day 7

Breakfast: Buckwheat pancakes with mixed berry compote, 1 cup of coffee

Optional Morning Snack: Corn and flaxseed tortilla chips, salsa

Lunch: Almond butter and jelly sandwich, vegetable soup

Optional Afternoon Snack: Wasabi peas

Dinner: Curry coleslaw salad, stuffed peppers with ground turkey, diced tomatoes, and rice

Dessert: Cottage cheese and pineapple

Reading List

Suggested Reading on Nutrition

If you're truly interested in exploring how to eat in a more healthy way I have created a list of great books on diet and nutrition written by authors with a knowledge base and credentials that are far superior to mine. Nutrition can be a very complicated subject and there are many different points of view on what's healthy and what's not. But there is no doubt that your overall health and wellbeing is directly tied to the foods you consume. It is my belief that in order to find your own right way to eat, it is important to educate yourself and then find a system that works for you and your personal tastes. Because, let's face it: if you hate the food you eat, you won't eat it for long no matter how good it is for you. I believe the books listed below can help you find a healthy way to eat and allow you to choose what best suits your lifestyle and taste. Bon Appétit!

The China Study, by T. Colin Campbell, Ph.D. & Thomas M. Campbell, II

Eat Your Way to Sexy, by Elizabeth Somer, M.A., R.D.

Real Food, by Nina Planck

What to Eat, by Luise Light, M.S., Ed.D.

Age-Proof Your Body, by Elizabeth Somer, M.A., R.D.

Staying Healthy with Nutrition, by Elson M. Hass, M.D. & Buck Levin, Ph.D., R.D.

The Paleo Diet, by Loren Cordain, Ph.D.

In Defense of Food, by Michael Pollan

The Okinawa Program, by Bradley J. Willcox M.D., D. Craig Willcox, Ph.D. & Makoto Suzuki, M.D.

The Raw Food Detox Diet, by Natalia Rose

The Omega Diet, by Artemis P. Simopoulos, M.D. & Joe Robinson

Good Calories Bad Calories, by Gary Taubes

Dr. Atkins New Diet Revolution, by Robert C. Atkins, M.D.

Exercise Sucks!

Chapter 3
It's the Little Things

The next step toward shedding those unwanted pounds is incorporating more regular movement into your daily life. This is probably the most difficult part of the plan, not because what I'm going to ask you to do requires great physical exertion or great feats of willpower, but because I'm going to ask you to override some very old habits. For most people, the movements we will talk about in this chapter are everyday activities. Most of them you probably never really think about, but these everyday activities are actually big calorie burners...or they can be. Our modern lifestyle and technology have pretty much sucked the calorie burn right out of our lives, which is why so many of us are overweight.

But how can it be true that the little things we do every day could actually be big calorie burners? If running for 30 minutes at a ten-minute-per-mile pace only burns 365 calories, how can the stuff I do during the course of my day possibly be considered a bigger calorie burn?

Well, it has to do with the law of frequency, or as I like to call it "The Sydney Effect." Sydney is my incredible daughter. She is the light of my life, she's beautiful and smart...very smart! And Sydney completely understands the law of frequency. Sydney knows, for example, that if she comes to me and asks for a largish sum of money, let's say $60, I will ask her what she needs it for (it's usually a "cute little top" or a pair of "drop dead gorgeous shoes"). Now, Sydney knows that getting me to hand over sixty bucks is like pulling teeth; it's a struggle she really doesn't want to deal with.

So instead, Sydney asks for $5. But it's not just a one-time occurrence. She asks for $5 twenty times over the course of the week. She sneaks up on me when I'm watching TV, she waits until her mother and I are deep in conversation, she asks while I'm cooking dinner. For me, $5 is painless and if I'm not paying attention, I forget that I gave it to her. With this simple strategy she knows she'll get that $60 plus a little extra for that great little skirt she's had her eye on. We can apply this same approach to our everyday activities. Most of us spend an average of 16 hours awake each day, so 20 calories here, 30 calories there, and the next thing you know you've burned seven or eight hundred extra calories over the course of just one day

Still don't believe me? Here are some real life numbers for you: A person who is chair-bound will burn roughly 300 calories above his or her Basal Metabolic Rate (BMR), or the amount of calories your body burns just staying alive. A person who sits at a desk job for most of the day, but gets up for lunch and a few water and restroom breaks, will burn roughly 700 calories over his or her BMR. A person who spends the majority of the day at a desk but manages to move around moderately (goes to the copier down the hall, makes several trips to the file room, walks to the water cooler) will burn 1000 calories over his or her BMR. The person whose job entails mostly standing or is very active will burn 1400 calories over his or her BMR, and the person who has a strenuous job, such as agricultural labor, can burn as much as 2,300 calories over his or her BMR. In order to lose one pound, you have to burn 3500 more calories than you take in. That basically boils down to burning 500 more calories a day to lose a pound a week, so you can see why being more active during the day makes it easier to lose weight.

On top of the simple calorie burn we get from increased activity, there is also a more complex biochemical process that happens on a cellular level. This process helps burn sugars and fats that can damage your metabolism, and an efficient, strong, and healthy metabolism keeps you slim and trim. All of this may seem very technical, but what I am basically saying is it is more than just calories in and calories out.

So what kinds of activities are we talking about? Actually, it's pretty mundane stuff. Included in this chapter is list of the things you can do to be more active. I suggest you pick one or two of the activities and try to concentrate on just those for a week or so, and then add one or two more per week after that. The reason for this slow build is that we do most of these mundane things on auto-pilot. Often you will find yourself halfway through the task before you even realize you started doing it, then you'll go: Dagnabit! I was supposed to stand up while I did that, Or some variation of that scenario (insert your favorite swear word). Keep in mind it will take some time to create these new habits, but these simple activities can be the key to your weight loss, so I want you to take this part of the process very seriously. Once you find yourself comfortably doing a new activity, move on to something else on the list.

In the next chapter I will offer some tools that will really help you to become more active, but the cool thing about this chapter is that everything is virtually *FREE.* Did I get your attention there?

-Place your alarm clock across the room so you have to walk over to shut it off

-Grind your coffee using an old fashioned hand grinder

-Eat breakfast standing up at the kitchen counter

-When listening to music in the car, tap your fingers on the steering wheel, shimmy your butt in the seat, and sing at the top of your lungs

-Park in the furthest parking space from your destination

-Place regularly used items in an area where you will have to get up to get them

-Always stand and pace when on the phone

-Fidget when sitting for more than twenty minutes (shake your legs, strum your fingers, twirl a pencil or pen)

-Create a stand up desk by placing a wide, sturdy cardboard box on top of your desk and place the keyboard and mouse on it. Use it every half hour.

-Have walking meetings with fellow workers

-Chew sugarless gum

-Drink small cups of water from the water cooler across the office so you'll have to make frequent trips

-Use the bathroom that is furthest from your desk

-Take the stairs instead of the elevator

-If your destination is less than a mile away, walk or ride your bike

Exercise Sucks!

-Make every coffee break a walking break

-Stand up and walk around the office every thirty minutes

-Deliver documents and messages to coworkers at their desk instead of calling or emailing

-Leave your lunch in the car or someplace you have to walk to get to it

-Chop vegetables instead of buying them pre-chopped

-Do the dishes by hand

-Run the vacuum over the entire house three times a day

-Fold clothes standing up

-Watch television while walking slowly (1-2 miles per hour) on a treadmill or pedaling a stationary bike

-If you sit watching television, get up and move during commercial breaks

-Walk the dog or take a 30 minute family stroll each evening

-Cut the grass with a push mower

-Shovel snow by hand (no snow blower)

-Do your own gardening

-Pace the sidelines during the kid's sporting events

-Have 30 minutes of *vigorous* sex each and every night (even if you're alone)

I'm sure you can think of more, but you get the idea. And I admit it: some of these things may seem a little silly, but I'm telling you *they work*. (Why do you think your bank charges all those little annoying fees? Because they add up to big money-- that's why!)

I'm not making this stuff up; there is science behind it. In 2005, Dr. Levine published a study that measured and compared the non-exercise activities of 10 men and women considered to be lean and 10 men and women considered to be slightly obese. All of the participants described themselves as being "couch potatoes" and none of them reported exercising much. The researchers conducting the study were attempting to determine whether the subjects' behaviors would change if they were put on special diets designed to make them gain or lose weight. The subjects wore specially designed underwear equipped with sensors that tracked their posture and every movement at half-second intervals around the clock, yielding as many as 25 million points of data on each participant. To make sure researchers collected accurate data, dietitians prepared each meal for the subjects, and every food item was weighed to be sure that every calorie each subject ate was counted.

The results of the study showed that the lean subjects spent much more time on their feet and were much more active than the obese subjects. Though it had been previously thought that, because they were heavy, extra weight made the obese subjects less active, the research showed that there was no difference in the activity levels of the obese subjects even when they lost weight; they were simply predisposed to being less active. Conversely, the subjects who had been lean and gained weight during the study were no less active, even though they had become heavier. In other words, the heavy people did not become more active when they lost weight and the lean people did not become less active when they gained weight. The findings of this study seem to suggest that our habits play a strong role in determining our activity and fitness levels. The good news is that all habits can be changed. It just takes time and patience and that, my friends, is exactly what I'm asking from you.

As with any new process, getting started can be the hardest part, so let's talk a little about how we can make some of this easier to do. By arranging your home or work station in such a way that you are forced to be more active changing your habits will become more a matter of necessity than conscious, effortful change. At the office, moving things you use on a regular basis, like staplers, calculators, and paper clips, to places that force you to get out of your seat to get them is an easy way to increase your activity. Putting file cabinets and the printer on the other side of the room is also helpful. So is not filling up a large water bottle for your desk, but instead going over to the water cooler when you get thirsty. At home a great idea is to set up a treadmill or stationary bike (you know, that thing you're currently using as a coat rack…) where you can see the television when you're on it. Instead of cranking that puppy up to a blistering pace that makes you feel nauseous just looking at it, set it at a nice, gentle setting, then watch a little TV, read a book or check out who's posting some great cat memes on Facebook or Pinterest. Now, perhaps you're thinking that all this extra moving around will make you less efficient throughout your day. Perhaps it will, but efficient and productive are two totally different things, and incorporating more activity into your day will actually help to make you more productive, more energetic, and more creative. Studies show that regular activity increases blood flow to the brain and has even been proven to make your brain grow. Most of us do things over the course of the day that are time wasters--things like organizing your desk, cleaning out your emails, making personal phone calls. These kinds of things allow us to gear up for concentrated attacks on the work we have to do. By replacing these sedentary breaks with active breaks we not only give your mind a chance to gather itself, we also feed it with nutrient- and oxygen-rich blood so that when you attack that report you are more focused, your ideas are more creative and your work is sharper than it would have been if you just sat at your desk. That's what I mean by productive.

If you find yourself having trouble turning over a new leaf, have no fear. There are some tools that can help. The next chapter will introduce these tools to you and get you all the help you need to get rid of those love handles and saddle bags.

Chapter 4

Tools

While they aren't necessities the following products can help give you a little extra boost toward getting your booty in gear or losing weight a little faster.

Stability Ball

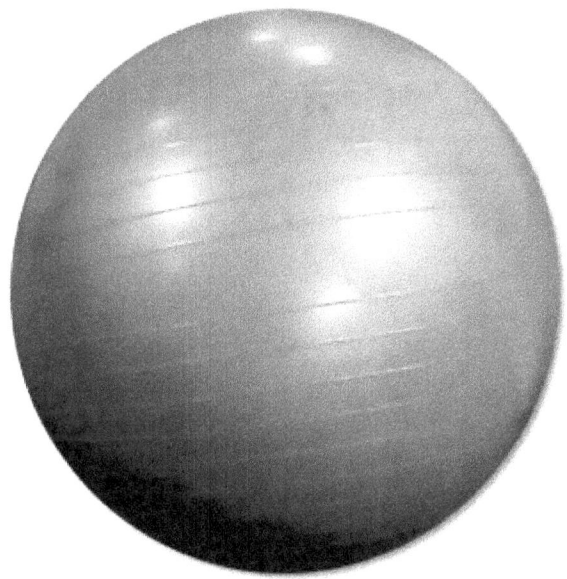

Stability balls have been around for decades. Typically, trainers use these to create instability in different exercises, forcing the body to use stabilizer muscles to improve strength and balance. When used as a chair, the stability ball forces you to activate your postural muscles to keep the ball from rolling away. The thigh muscles are also much more active on the ball than on a traditional chair, and for people who are fidgety like me, the ball offers unlimited opportunities to move around. The stability ball will help you burn a lot more calories than you would if you just sat in a regular chair all day. The major downside to the stability ball is that it's pretty easy to fall off of, which can be a bit embarrassing at the office. Stability Balls range in price from $13.00 to $60.00 depending on size, quality, and how much weight they can support.

http://astore.amazon.com/kenbur-20

Stand-Up Desk

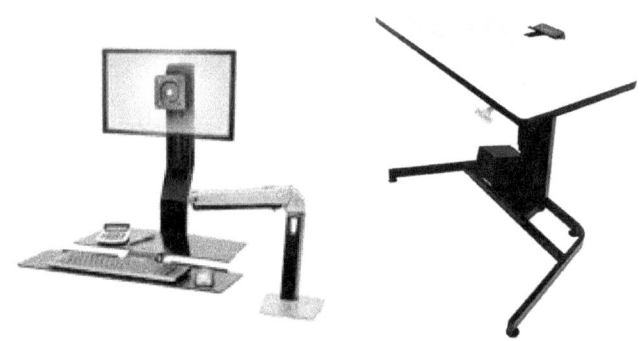

WorkFit S   **WorkFit D Sit/Stand Desk**

Of all the tools to help you burn more calories during the work day the stand up desk is my favorite. While I don't recommend standing all day long (there are some studies that show standing all day increases the risk of varicose veins) standing for 30 minutes and sitting 20 minutes keeps me energized without the tired feet and legs I sometimes get with standing alone. And the health, weight loss, and improved energy benefits are outstanding. Most stand-up desks are desks that are taller than traditional desks and therefore meant to be stood at. These are not new. In fact, author Ernest Hemingway was said to use a stand-up desk, as was Secretary of Defense Donald Rumsfeld. Standing desks take a little getting used to, but most people rave about their standing desks after the adjustment period. Mostly you hear about weight loss, disappearing back pain, and increasing energy levels.

My favorite stand up desk is made by Ergotron and is pictured above. The reason I like it is that it's not a conventional stand up desk. It's actually is a combo sit-stand desk (like the one pictured above) that effortlessly moves from a sitting to a standing position whenever you want. The desk I use is customized with accessories to fit individual users' needs and workflow. It has effortless height adjustment that is instantaneous and tool-free, so you can do it while you work! The large sit stand desk runs about $900.00. Ergotron also offers a WorkFit Station that attaches to your current desk and adjust to your height as you sit or stand (it's also pictured above). Usually these include an adjustable arm that allows you to move the keyboard and the monitor out of the way when you don't need them. These attachable work stations also give you the flexibility to move from sitting to standing in just seconds, and best of all is the price! While a sit-stand desk can cost around $900, attachable work stations go for around just $495. I have also seen several money-saving designs, such as putting desks up on boxes, and placing monitors and keyboards on flat boards resting on full cases of canned soft drinks, though getting the ergonomics just right can be challenging. Don't be afraid to think outside the box; this is one of those cases where a little imagination can get you a healthier workspace for very little money

http://astore.amazon.com/kenbur-20

Stationary Bike Desk

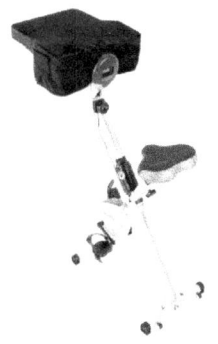

Figure FitDesk Stationary Bike Desk

I really like the Fitdesk stationary bike desk because using it involves activating a large number of the big muscle groups and the smaller postural muscle groups, the calorie burn is significant. It also has the advantage of being really safe, even for those with very little body awareness (that's a polite term for people like my wife, which is to say *a little klutzy*). They are safe because falling off the bike is far less likely to occur if you get distracted by a call or email and forget to move your feet (which has been known to happen on treadmill desks).What makes this different from an ordinary stationary bike is its low intensity setting which won't leave you sweaty at the office and its ability to easily and securely hold your lap top computer and a bottle of water. The other thing that makes it both office and home friendly is its ability to fold up and be put away into a small space.

http://astore.amazon.com/kenbur-20

Under Desk Pedal Machines

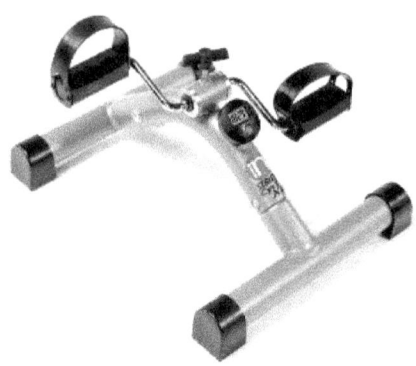

InStride Cycle XL

Under-desk pedal machines are simple and effective, but above all they are inexpensive! Starting at $30.00 and going up to the low $100.00 range, these little babies store easily and no one even needs to know they're there. The calorie burn isn't huge but it's certainly better than just sitting in your chair doing nothing. The other great thing about these units is their complete portability. You can take them to the office then grab them as you head home to use in front of the TV.

http://astore.amazon.com/kenbur-20

Treadmill Desks

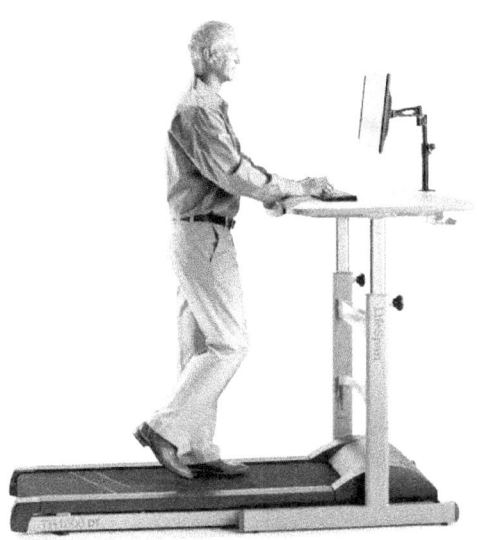

TR 1200-DT Treadmill Desk Combination

This type of treadmill desk is Dr. Levine's secret weapon. According to his book *Move a Little Lose a Lot*, with the addition of this single tool he lost 30 pounds. A treadmill desk is the Rolls Royce of weight-loss office/home furniture from a calorie-burning and postural-muscle-engaging standpoint—it's also the most expensive option. These desks combine exactly what our body was created to do, walking, with the ease of use that a traditional desk offers. Heck, several models even actually incorporate cup holders in the design! The walking pace can be controlled so that you don't feel overwhelmed or get sweaty. The work space can be raised or lowered for ultimate comfort and the potential daily calorie burn is huge. The learning curve for most people is about 3 hours, but after that, the term I've heard most often used to describe the experience is "addictive." The secret seems to be to find the perfect speed for you. Too slow and you can't find a rhythm. Too fast and you'll feel like you're going to fall off while you do your basic daily tasks. But once you find your sweet spot, it's like nirvana. In addition to the physical benefits, most researchers noted better brain function and an increase in alertness and focus throughout the day. Personally, I know that I think more clearly and get more done when I'm walking. In fact, I tend to do my best work while on the move, so the walking desk fits me to a tee. If you're interested in walking and working at the same time you have a couple of different options. If you don't currently have a treadmill, one option is to buy a treadmill that has a desk integrated or attached to it. Traditional treadmills aren't really designed for day in and day out use at low speeds, so if you plan to use this equipment daily, then a complete system like the one pictured above may be a wiser purchase.

However, if you already own a treadmill you can always just buy a desk for it, like the TrekDesk (pictured below). This type of product is specifically designed to simply fit over the treadmill you already own.

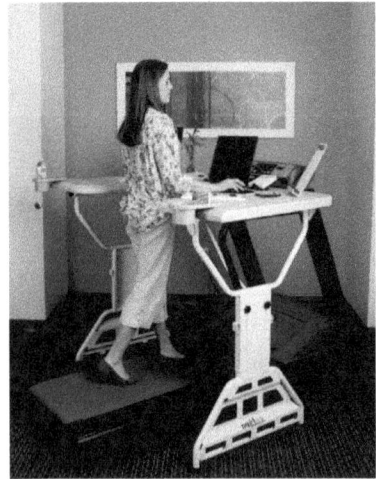

TrekDesk Treadmill Desk

I accomplished a similar set up myself with some power tools and a little elbow grease (though in all fairness, mine is pretty ghetto-looking and doesn't have anywhere near the work surface area or cool cup holders).

Pedometers

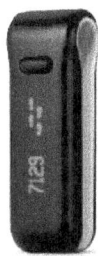

FitBit Ultra Wireless Activity Plus Sleep Tracker

Pedometers can be a great tool to help you stay on track as you navigate through the process of increasing your activity level. But be aware that pedometers vary in quality, accuracy, and price. The reason I'm a big pedometer fan is that it takes a lot of the guess work out of figuring out just how active you are over the course of the day. In my experience, most people overestimate how active they are.

My personal favorite is the Fitbit Ultra Wireless Activity Plus Sleep Tracker pictured above. Now, the Fitbit is not cheap-- about a hundred bucks. But it does so much! It accurately tracks daily steps, stairs climbed, distance, calories burned, and activity level via 3-d motion sensor and altimeter technology. It can measures how long and how well you sleep - just wear it on your wrist at night with the Fitbit wristband. It's small and discreet enough to wear all day (you can just tuck it into a pocket or clip it to a belt or bra). The thing wirelessly uploads data to Fitbit.com with no monthly fee and you can see online graphs, compete with friends, earn nifty badges, log food consumption, weight changes and workout-related info at Fitbit.com and on the iPhone app.

http://astore.amazon.com/kenbur-20

Again, these tools can help you be successful and speed up your weight loss, but keep in mind that you don't need to own all of them to start a successful fitness routine. Picking up all the stuff in this chapter could send you down the road to the poor house, so just choose wisely, and take into account your own individual needs, challenges, and budget.

Exercise Sucks!

Chapter 5

Caution: These Movements are
(Keystone) Habit Forming

Now you've rearranged your office and the house is all set up for your new more active lifestyle. It's time to take the next step and the next step is going to change everything. How you say? Well, my friends, it all comes down to our habits. In his bestselling book *The Power of Habit: Why We Do What We Do In Life And Business*, Charles Duhigg identifies what are known as "keystone habits." A keystone habit is a small, simple change in behavior that is easy to do and repeat. As this small positive habit becomes a part of your life you develop a sense of accomplishment. This small positive habit leads to other positive habits creating a domino-effect in your life. According to Duhigg, "Most people think of a habit as a routine, but it's actually a cue, a routine, and a reward."

In other words, by focusing on just one pattern a person can make huge shifts in the things they do and the way they do them. This is exactly what we will be doing as we change how you do the things you do over the course of your day to override the old sitting habit and introduce new healthier patterns.

To start this process we have developed a series of movements that we will turn into "keystone habits." What make these keystone habits so powerful is they are easy to accomplish, yet make us feel like we are making meaningful changes. This in turn makes us want to make more meaningful changes in our lives, which starts a domino effect. It's sort of like deciding to paint your kitchen cabinets. After you do the painting you feel like you did something positive for the way the kitchen looks, but then you notice that the counter top looks a little drab now that the cabinets look so good, so you replace the counter tops. After replacing the counter tops, now the appliances are looking a little dated... you get the picture.

In order to make these movements part of your daily habits you will have to do three things: First, you will need to create a cue, which you can do on your own with an alarm or timer. Set up the alarm or timer to go off at about the same time every hour (i.e. at the top of the hour or quarter after the hour, whatever is right for you).You may not be able to stand up and move at that exact time, but you will start to anticipate it and build the expectation and the habit. To help you get started, my company is developing software that shows you the movements as well as reminds you to do them, and has a host of other features as well including some pretty cool rewards. You can find out more about it at www.mylifefitness.com.

Second, you will need to do the movements when you are cued. This can be more effective if this happens at a regular time each day but I know that few of us have the kind of days that we can count on any given time to be convenient. Third, and finally, you will need to reward yourself for sticking with your new habit. Here's one cautionary note: try not to reward yourself for doing the movements with fatty or sugary treats as this can nullify all the good work you do.

These simple movements based on yoga, Pilates, tai chi, and physical therapy can be done at your desk or almost anywhere. They won't make you break a sweat but will get you up and moving.

These movements should be done for 3-5 minutes every hour. Choose several of the movements to do every hour depending on how long each movement is done.

You will notice that the menu of movements is broken up into four categories: Flexibility, Energy, Balance and Strength. Choose two or three movements from each category or choose movements based on what your personal needs are for that particular hour. Maybe you are thinking "I feel like I could fall asleep right now, I should do some energizing movements," or "Ryan's secretary usually passes by my cubicle for her break about this time every day—I think I'll do a few strength movements and pump up a little bit!"

These simple movements will start the process of leading you down the road to losing the weight you want to lose and help you feel and look better than you ever have before.

Menu of Movements

As you go through the movement section of this book and try out the movements, keep in mind that breathing is very important. In other words: Don't hold your breath! It is important to keep breathing throughout the entire time that you are doing these movements.

Throughout this section, movement descriptions appear **above** the pictures that illustrate that movement.

Flexibility Movements

Chair-Supported Downward Facing Dog

Rise from seated position and walk behind chair. Secure chair so it will not move or roll away. Facing back of chair, grab top of chair back and take a step or two backwards away from chair until arms are fully extended. Hinge at hips and lean forward, bringing torso parallel to floor beneath you. You should feel a gentle stretch in low back and hamstring muscles. Hold for 30 seconds.

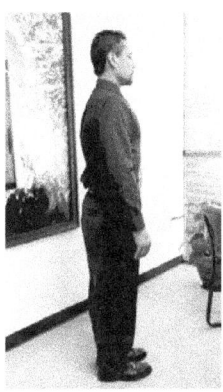 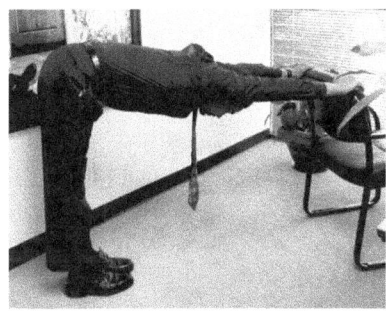

Modified Hanging Pose

Begin in a standing position with feet hip distance apart. Bend both knees slightly, then lean forward and slowly lower head as you begin to reach down toward mid-thighs or knees, depending on what feels comfortable for you. Support upper body with hands, and allow spine to lengthen toward floor as much as feels comfortable. Hold pose for 5 long, slow, deep breaths.

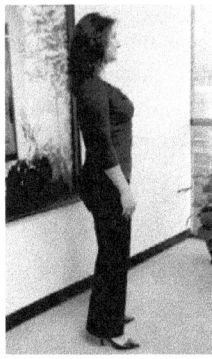 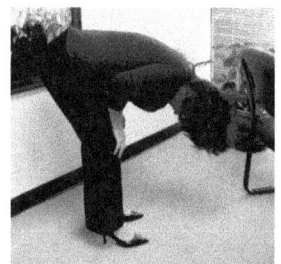

Turning the Head

Begin in a standing position with arms hanging at sides and palms of hands facing body. *Very slowly* turn head to the right and look over right shoulder, rotating palms so they point out and away from body. *Very slowly* turn head back so you are looking forward again and rotate palms back toward body. *Very slowly* turn head to the left and look over left shoulder as you rotate palms out and away from body. *Very slowly* turn head back to starting position and rotate palms back toward body again.

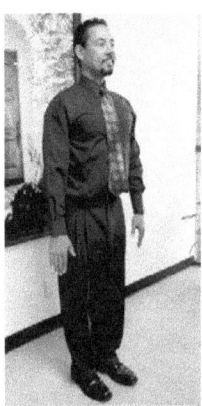 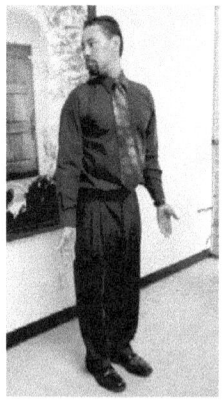

Baby Camel Prays to the Gods

From a standing position place hands on front of thighs for support, then lean forward as you roll shoulders inward, rounding back and dropping chin down to chest to create a humped back. Pause for a moment, and then one vertebra at a time bring yourself back up to a standing position, bringing arms down to sides. Slowly roll shoulders back, lift chest, and look to sky.

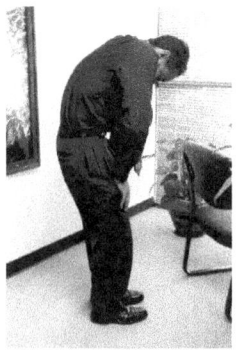 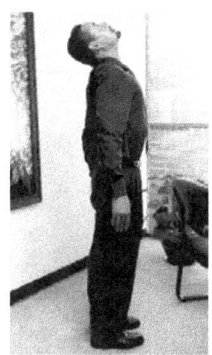

Hip Swivels

Stand with feet hip distance apart. Place hands on hips and slowly start to roll hips in a circle. Make circles a little bigger with each swivel of hips. After 10 seconds, switch directions.

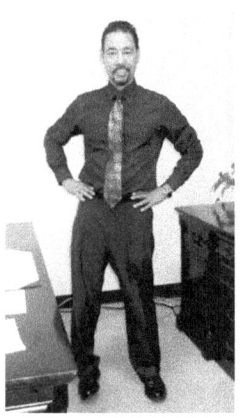 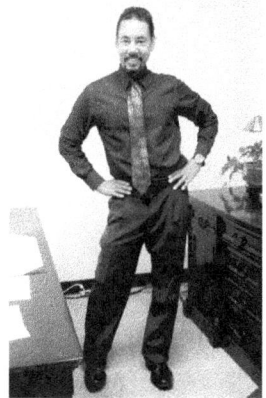

Shoulder Rolls

Stand with feet hip distance apart, arms hanging down at sides. Gently roll shoulders forward, down, and back, making as big a circle with shoulders as you comfortably can. After 5 or 10 seconds, reverse direction of circles.

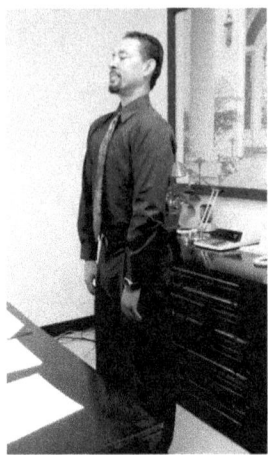 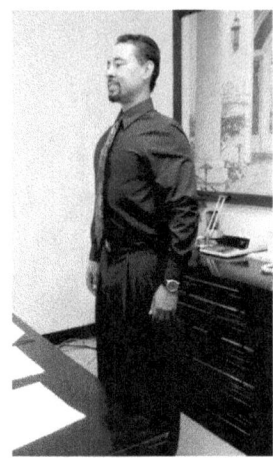

Neck Rolls

Stand with feet hip distance apart, arms hanging down at sides. Gently roll head in small circles then slowly make each circle a little bigger. After 5 or 10 seconds, reverse direction of circles.

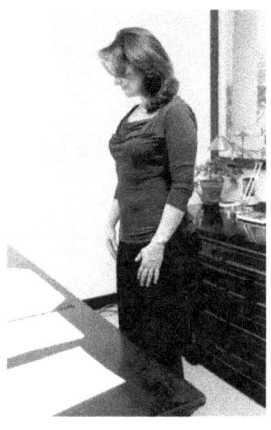 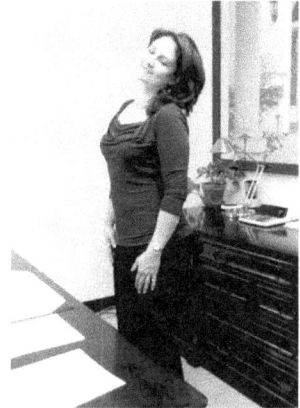

Pec (pectoral) Stretch

From a standing position bring both hands together behind back and interlace fingers. Press chest out as you lift joined hands upward, towards backs of shoulders. Hold for 10 seconds.

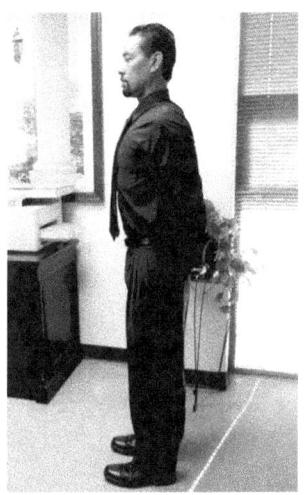 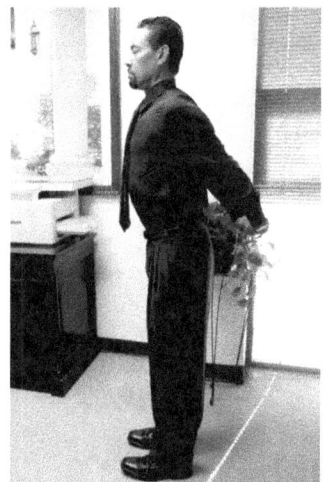

Quad & Hip Flexor Stretch

Stand and hold onto a chair or desk with left hand. Bend right knee, bringing right heel up towards buttocks. Reach down and grab right ankle. Pull kneecap down towards floor and press right hip gently forward. Hold for 5 to 10 seconds. Switch sides.

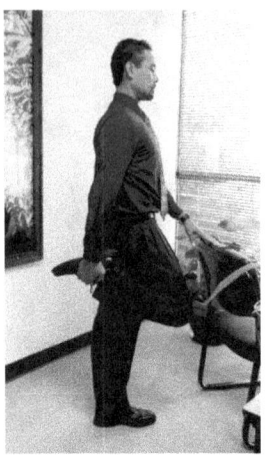 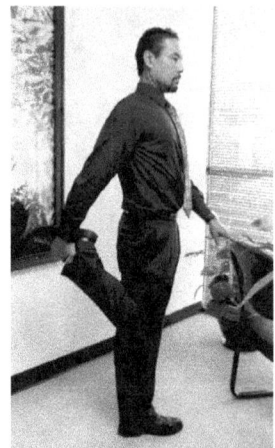

Calf Stretch

From a standing position, turn and face a desk or wall. Place palms of hands on desk or wall and bend left knee slightly, stepping back with right foot. Press heel down towards ground and lean gently forward. You should feel a gentle stretch at back of lower right leg. Hold for 5 to 10 seconds, then switch legs.

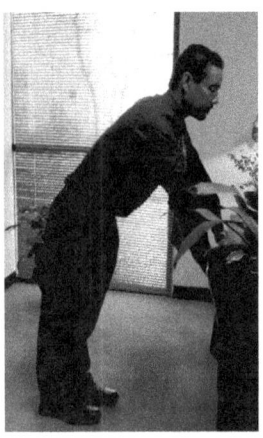 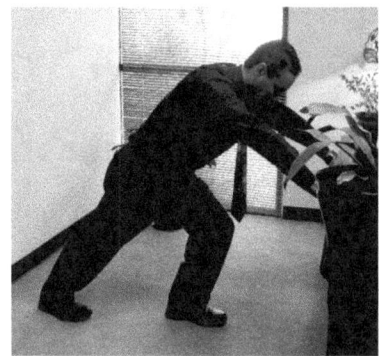

Half Eagle

You can do this one from either a standing or seated position. Bring left arm directly out in front of you at chest level. Bend elbow and point forearm and hand up towards sky. Take right arm and cross right bicep under left elbow, reaching with right hand up and around left forearm and grabbing inside of left wrist. Hold for 5 to 10 seconds, then switch sides.

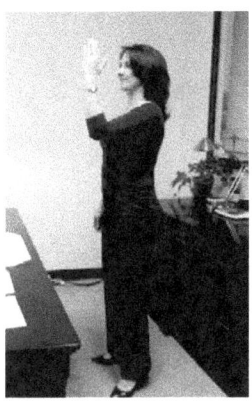 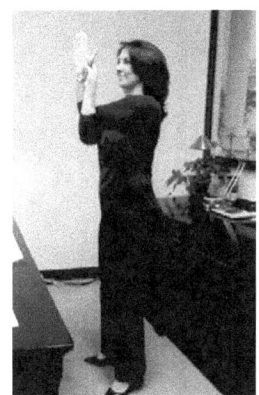

Triceps Stretch

You can do this one from either a standing or seated position. Reach up towards ceiling with right arm, then drop right hand down behind head, pointing right elbow up towards ceiling. Reach up to right elbow with left hand and gently pull elbow towards midline of body until you feel a gentle stretch in back of right tricep. Hold for 5 to 10 seconds, then switch arms.

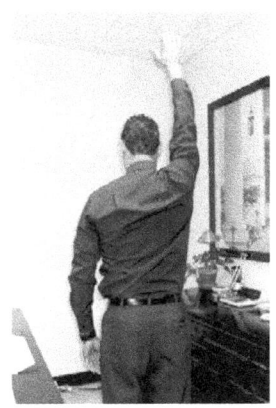 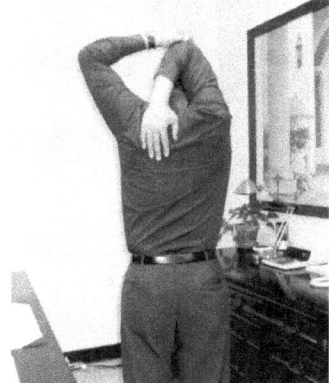

Hamstring Stretch

From a standing position, step forward approximately 2 feet with right foot, keeping right knee straight but not locked. Hinge at hips, leaning forward until you feel a gentle stretch in back of right thigh. Hold for 5 to 10 seconds, then switch legs.

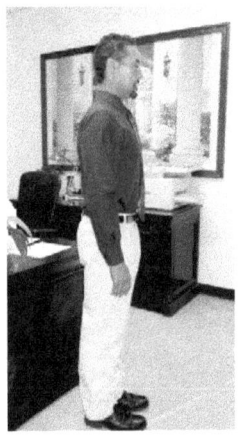
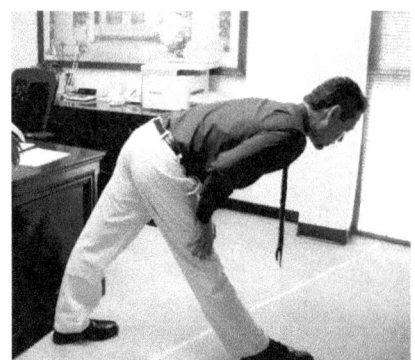

Side-Step Lunge

Begin in a standing position with feet hip distance apart. Step about 12 inches to the right with right foot. Keep left knee straight and bend right knee, leaning out towards right foot until you feel a gentle stretch on inside of left leg. Hold for 5 to 10 seconds, then switch sides.

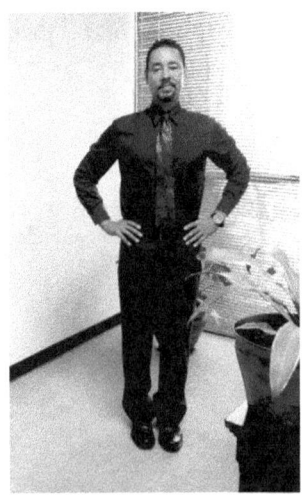
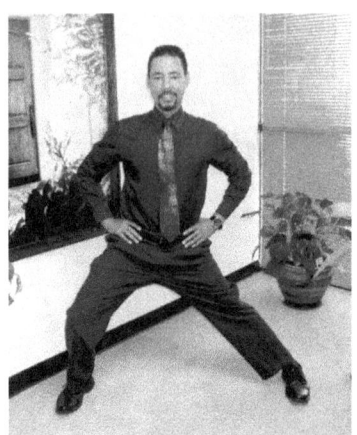

The Archway

Begin by standing in front of a stable desk or chair. Turn back to desk or chair and place palms of hands on desk or chair behind you, with fingers pointed away from body. Keeping hands on desk or chair, take a short step away with both feet, then arch back and press chest up towards ceiling. Gently drop head back and look up at ceiling. Hold for 10 seconds, then walk feet back to starting position.

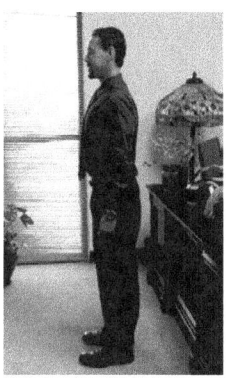 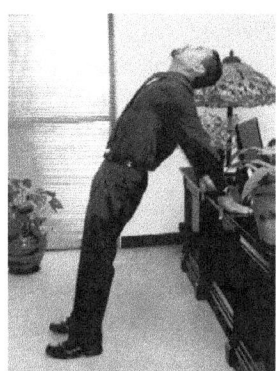

Round and Open

Sitting in a chair with feet on floor, begin by bringing shoulders directly above hips, lengthening spine upward, head floating away from shoulders. Drop chin down to chest and slowly lean forward as you roll shoulders in towards chest, making an exaggerated hump in back. Bring forearms to fronts of thighs as you pull shoulder blades apart. Hold for 30 seconds as you breathe.

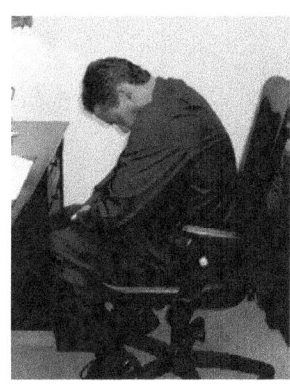 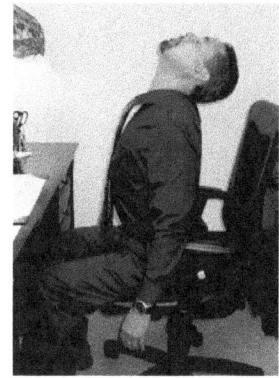

Now, slowly, one vertebra at a time, bring yourself back up to a tall seated position, then roll shoulders back, open chest, arch back and look up to ceiling. Breathe deeply as you let arms drop down to sides. Hold for 30 seconds, then return to tall seated position.

Seated Forward Fold (you don't have to get up for this one either!)

Begin in a tall seated position with feet about hip distance apart. Hinge at hips as you lean forward from waist. Drape front of torso over front of thighs, dropping head between knees and grabbing hold of ankles. Let head drop and dangle, relaxing neck. Pull lower spine away from hips. You should feel a gentle stretch in lower- and mid-back. Hold for 30 seconds, then return to tall seated position.

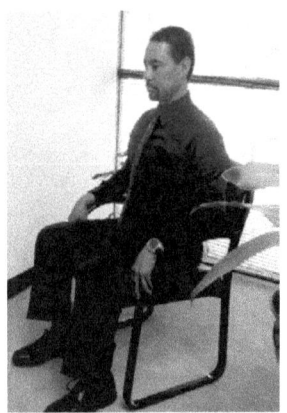 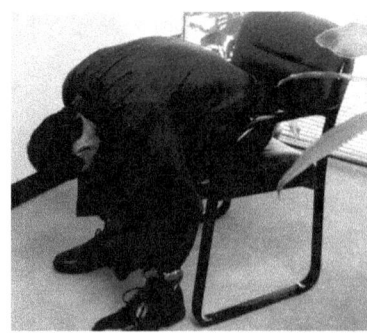

Sitting Man-Style

Begin in a tall seated position. Cross right ankle over left knee, creating a triangle shape with right leg, then gently press down on inside of right knee until you feel a gentle stretch through hip and buttocks. Hold for 30 seconds. Now, gently lean forward, bringing chest down towards legs; this should intensify the stretch. Hold for another 30 seconds. Switch sides and repeat on other side, then return to tall seated position.

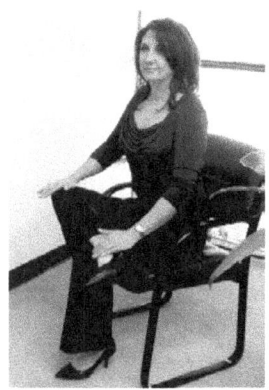 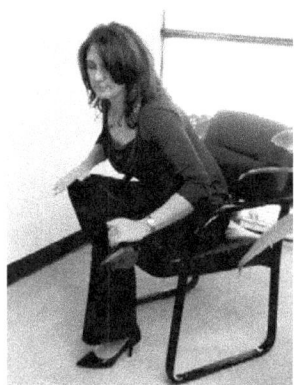

Seated Twist

Begin in a tall seated position. With both feet on floor, gently turn to the right, keeping spine long yet relaxed. With right arm, reach to back of chair and twist torso, using back of chair for leverage. Without straining neck, turn head and torso as if you were going to look behind you. Hold for 30 seconds. Repeat on opposite side, then return to tall seated position.

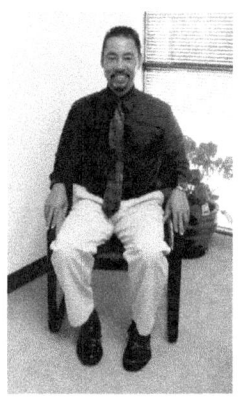 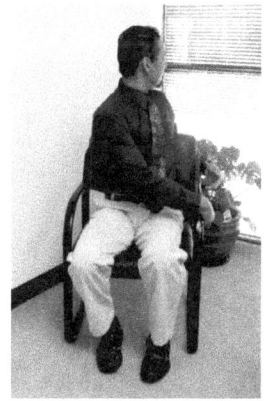

Cross Legged Seated Twist

Begin in a tall seated position. Cross right leg tightly over left leg (as if you were wearing a short skirt or kilt). Gently turn to the right, keeping spine long yet relaxed. With right arm, reach to back of chair and twist torso, using back of chair for leverage. With left hand, gently press knees towards left side of chair. Without straining neck, turn head and torso as if you were going to look behind you. Hold for 30 seconds. Repeat on opposite side, then return to tall seated position.

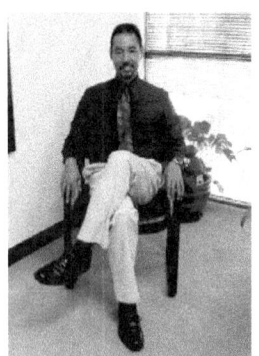 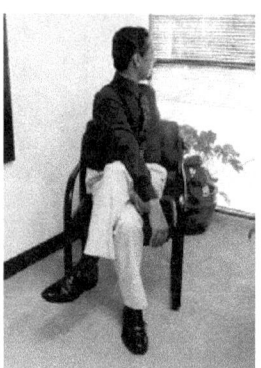

Balance Movements

All of these movements can be done while steadying yourself on an immovable object.

Wu Chi Stance

Stand with feet slightly wider than hip distance apart. Bend knees slightly (the deeper you bend knees, the more challenging this exercise becomes). Now tuck tailbone under spine, lengthening lower back. Let arms dangle at sides. Roll shoulders gently open and relax chest. Allow head to float off shoulders. Hold for 30 seconds.

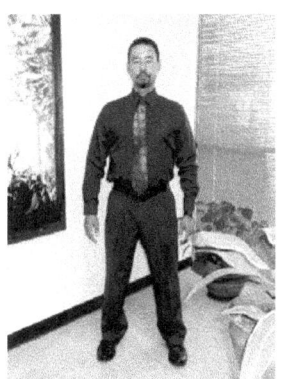 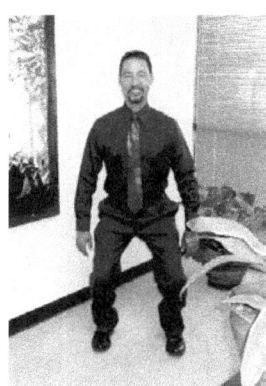

Dog Wags His Tail (Modified)

From Wu Chi Stance, bring hands down to fronts of thighs and rest them there. Bend knees a little deeper and lower back long, keeping tailbone tucked under spine. Now slowly shift weight over to right foot and pause there for a moment (for more of a challenge, lift left heel off ground with only toe touching).Then with both feet firmly on ground again, shift weight over to left foot and pause for a moment (you can lift right heel if you wish). Go back and forth between the two feet 3 or 4 times.

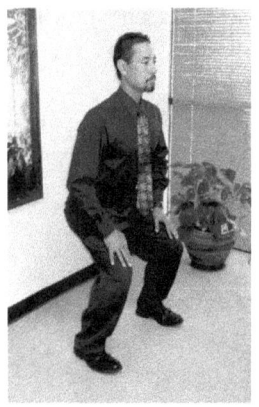 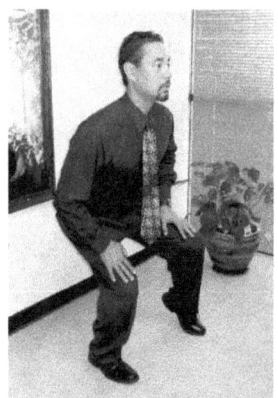

Sumo Step

Stand with legs twice hip width apart. Drop buttocks down 6 to 10 inches, bringing you into a wide-legged squat position (the deeper the squat the more challenging this becomes). Shift weight over to right foot and slowly lift left foot off ground 1 to 8 inches. Hold for a count of 5, then slowly lower left foot back to ground. Repeat on opposite side.

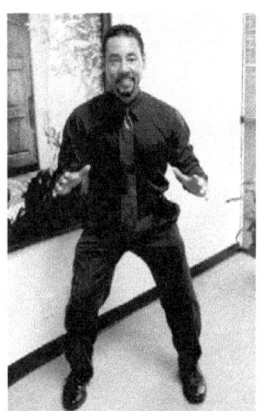 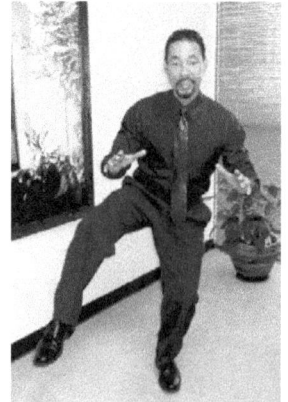

Ankle Circles

Stand with feet hip distance apart. Shift weight onto left foot and slowly lift right foot off ground. Balance on left foot for a breath or two, then slowly roll right foot in a circle for 5 seconds. Slowly bring right foot back down to ground and repeat with left foot.

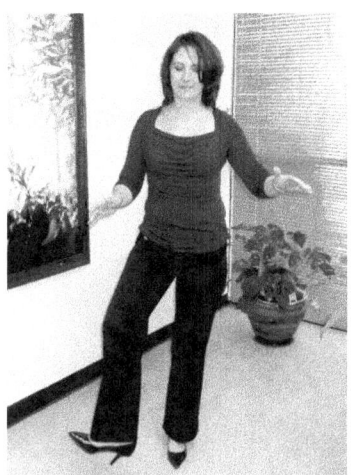 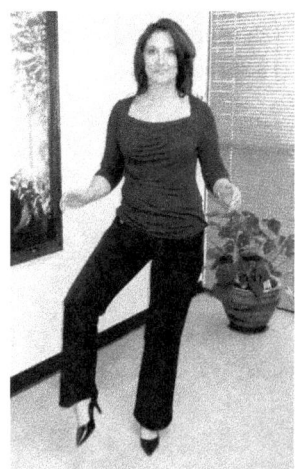

Lifting the Knee

Stand with feet hip distance apart. Shift weight onto left foot and slowly lift right foot off ground. Bring knee up slowly until it is even with hip (thigh should be parallel to floor), then slowly lower it back down to floor. Switch legs and repeat.

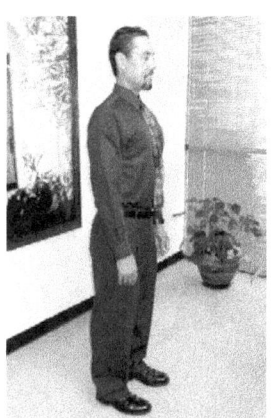 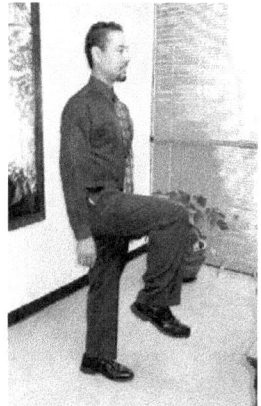

Empty Step

Stand with feet hip distance apart. Shift weight onto left foot and slowly lift right foot off ground. Bring knee up slowly until it is even with hip. Extend right foot and bend left knee, touching toe of right foot on floor about 12 inches in front of you, putting no weight on right foot (as if you were testing water temperature in a lake you were thinking of swimming in). Lift knee back up to hip level, then return to starting position. Switch legs and repeat.

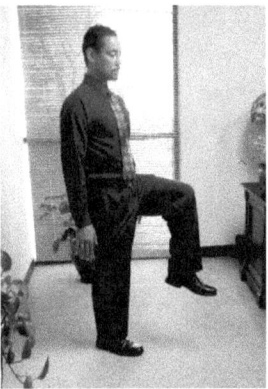 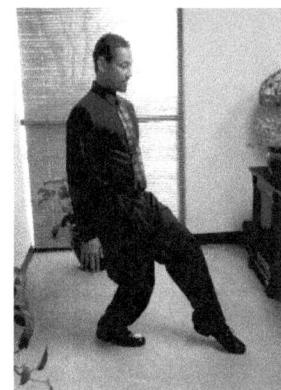

Raising your Internal Temperature

Stand with feet hip distance apart. Begin to march in place very slowly, raising right leg to a slow count of 3 then lowering it to a slow count of 3, then do the same with left foot. Continue alternating for 10 to 20 seconds.

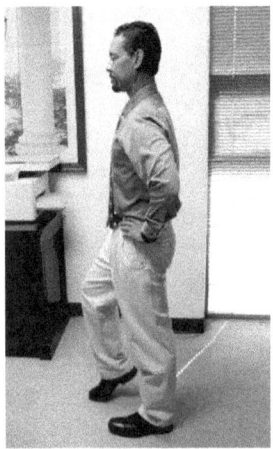 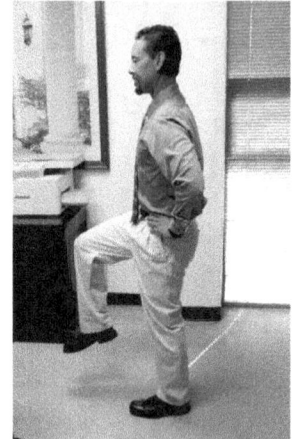

Tree Pose (modified)

Stand with feet hip distance apart. Shift weight onto left foot and bring right foot off ground. Place sole of right foot against calf of left leg. Bring palms of hands together in prayer position in middle of chest, then forcefully push them together. Hold for 10 seconds, then switch legs.

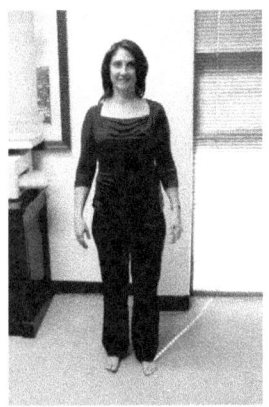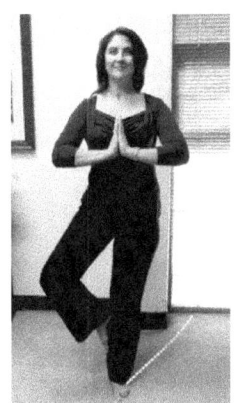

Standing Single Leg Circles

Standing to the right of an immovable desk or chair, begin with feet hip distance apart. Place left hand on a desk or chair to steady yourself, then shift weight onto left foot, keeping torso erect and spine tall. Lift right leg out to side, pointing toe at floor (foot should be about 6 inches off floor). Make a circle about the size of a volleyball with foot for 10 seconds. Switch sides and repeat.

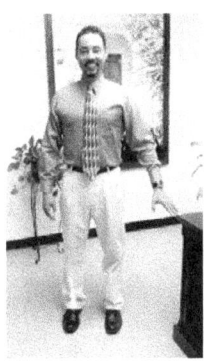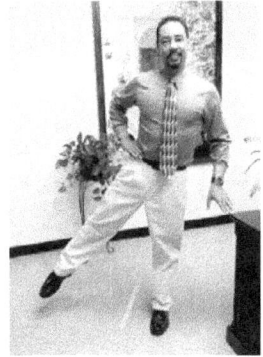

61

Standing Single Leg Back Beats

Standing to the right of a steady desk or chair, begin with feet hip distance apart. Place left hand on desk or chair to steady yourself, then shift weight onto left foot, keeping torso erect and spine tall. Lift right leg backwards, pointing toe. Lift foot anywhere from 1 to 12 inches off floor (the higher you lift the leg, the more difficult the movement). Drop foot down to floor and lightly touch toe on ground, then lift it again. Repeat for 10 seconds, then switch sides.

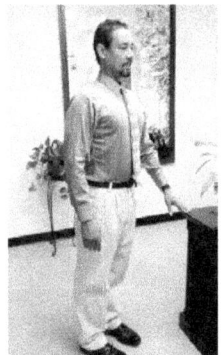 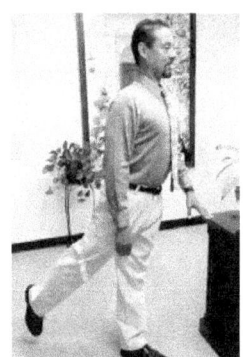

Standing Single Leg Side Beats

Standing to the right of a steady desk or chair, begin with feet hip distance apart. Place left hand on desk or chair to steady yourself then shift weight onto left foot, keeping torso erect and spine tall. Lift right leg sideways (out to the right of body) as you point toe. Lift foot anywhere from 1 to 12 inches off floor (the higher you lift the leg the more difficult the movement). Drop foot down to floor and lightly touch toe on ground, then lift it again. Repeat for 10 seconds, then switch sides.

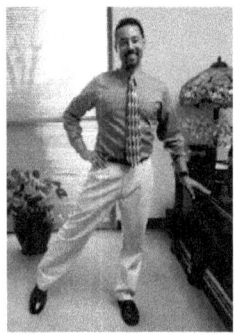 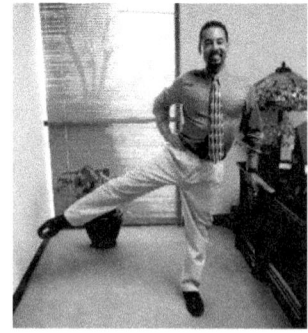

Standing Single Leg Front Beats

Standing to the right of a steady desk or chair, begin with feet hip distance apart. Place left hand on desk or chair to steady yourself, then shift weight onto left foot, keeping torso erect and spine tall. Lift right leg forward (out in front of body) as you point toe. Lift foot anywhere from 1 to 12 inches off floor (the higher you lift the leg the more difficult the movement). Drop foot down to floor and lightly touch toe on ground, then lift it again. Repeat for 10 seconds, then switch sides.

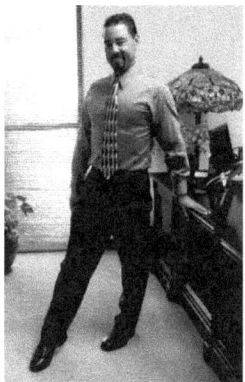 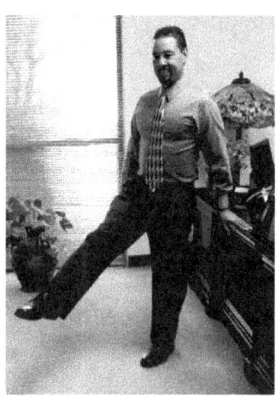

Energizing Movements

Lifting the Sky

Bring hands up in front of hips, palms facing up as if you were supporting a large belly in front of you. Slowly pull palms up towards chin, keeping hands a few inches away from front of body. When hands reach chest, rotate palms down, forward, and up until palms face sky, then press upward until arms are extended overhead, as if lifting sky. When arms are fully extended overhead allow them to swing outward in a wide arc to sides, coming slowly back to starting position.

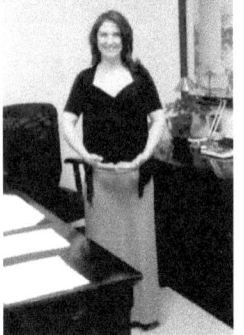 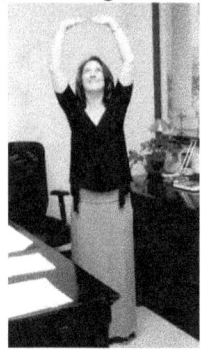

Shake Illness from the Body

Begin in a standing position, feet hip distance apart, arms hanging at sides of body. Lift up onto toes as high as you can and pause. Drop down heavily on soles of feet and shake body and arms vigorously (if this brings you pain simply drop down gently, minimizing the bang at the bottom). Repeat 3 to 4 times.

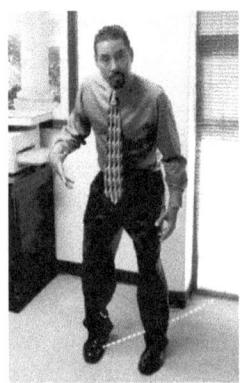 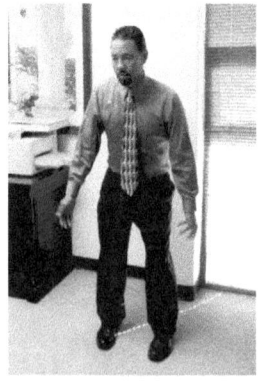

Awakening the Chi

From a standing position with feet hip distance apart, bend knees slightly. Inhale deeply through nose, then slowly exhale out through mouth. Continue to breathe like this the entire time you do the rest of the movements. Take hands and begin to slap fronts of thighs vigorously. You should feel area being slapped begin to feel tingly; if it hurts, you're slapping too hard. Move to backs of thighs, then up to buttocks. Move up body slapping fronts of hips, belly, chest, shoulders, arms, and finally face.

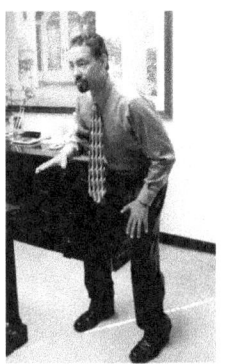 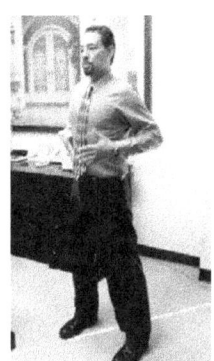

Opening the Door

Stand with feet slightly wider than hip distance apart. Bend knees slightly (the deeper you bend the knees the more challenging this movement becomes). Now tuck tailbone under spine, lengthening lower back. Let arms dangle at sides. Roll shoulders gently open and relax chest. Allow head to float off shoulders. Inhale deeply through nose as you slowly raise arms in front of you, palms facing down towards ground, muscles relaxed and soft, until arms reach shoulder height. Raise palms so they face forward, and exhale through mouth as you slowly lower arms back down to starting position. Repeat 5 times.

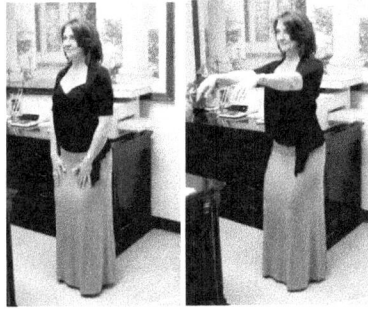

Two Full Moons

Stand with feet slightly wider than hip distance apart. Bend knees slightly (the deeper you bend the knees, the more challenging this exercise becomes). Now tuck tailbone under spine, lengthening lower back. Let arms dangle at sides. Roll shoulders gently open and relax chest. Allow head to float off shoulders. Inhale deeply through nose as you slowly raise arms in front of you, palms facing down towards ground, muscles relaxed and soft, until arms are up over head. Swing both arms out to sides as you exhale and lower arms back down to sides. Repeat 5 times.

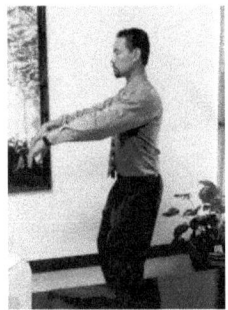 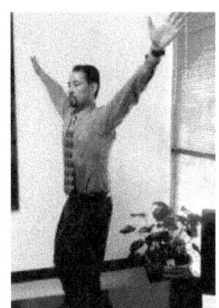

Swimming on Land

Stand with feet slightly wider than hip distance apart. Bend knees slightly (the deeper you bend the knees, the more challenging this exercise becomes). Now tuck tailbone under spine, lengthening lower back. Bring hands up in front of chest, elbows pointing outward. Start to move hands as if you were doing the breast stroke (a wide circular motion at chest height). Inhale deeply through nose and exhale slowly through mouth as you continue to "swim" with arms. Do this for 5 breaths.

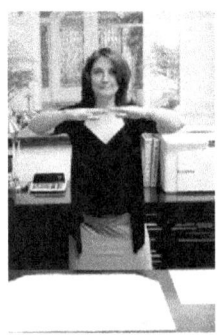 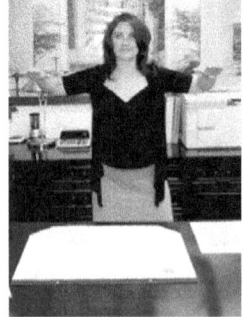

Bending Backwards

Stand with feet slightly wider than hip distance apart. Now tuck tailbone under spine, lengthening lower back. Place both hands behind you at small of back and gently lean backwards. As you begin to lean back, bend knees slightly and press hips forward. Allow chest to rise upward as you look up at ceiling. Hold for 1 to 2 seconds, then return to starting position. Repeat 5 times.

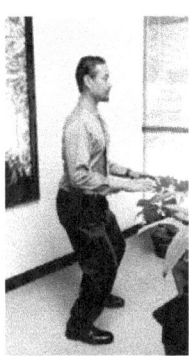 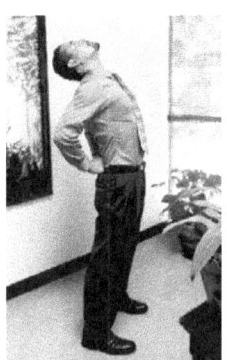

Bending to the sides

Stand with feet slightly wider than hip distance apart. Place right hand on right hip. Bring left hand up over head as you gently lean to the right, pressing left hip out to the left. Reach with left hand over head until you feel a gentle stretch all along left side. Hold for 5 to 10 seconds, then switch sides.

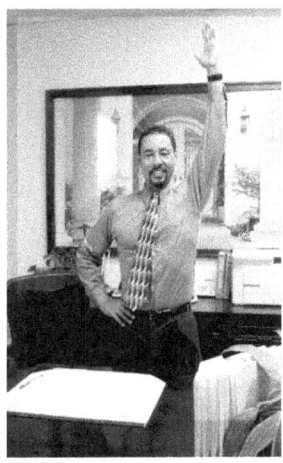 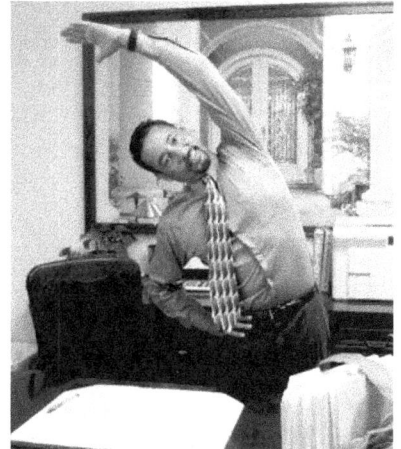

Looking back at the moon

Stand facing forward with feet slightly wider than hip distance apart. Place both hands on hips and slowly twist at waist as you turn entire upper body to the left. Be sure to keep feet firmly planted on floor. Turn head to the left as if looking behind you and hold for 5 seconds. Switch sides.

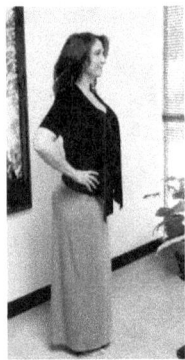 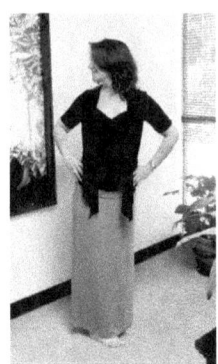

Strength Movements

A note on breathing during the strength movements: Try to exhale during the harder phase of each movement and inhale during the easier part of each movement.

Pulling the Bow

Stand with feet slightly wider than hip distance apart. Swing elbows outward as you bring hands up to chest, palms facing body. Ball hands into fists (tops of fists should be facing one another). The next movement is like an archer pulling his bow: keeping left hand where it is, slowly extend right arm out to right side at shoulder height as if ready to the shoot an arrow. Hold for a moment, feeling the tension between bow and string. Slowly bring right hand back to chest. Keep right hand were it is and slowly extend left arm out to left side at shoulder height as if ready to shoot an arrow. Hold for a moment, feeling the tension between bow and string. Slowly bring left hand back to chest.

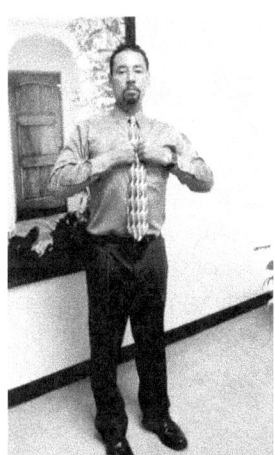 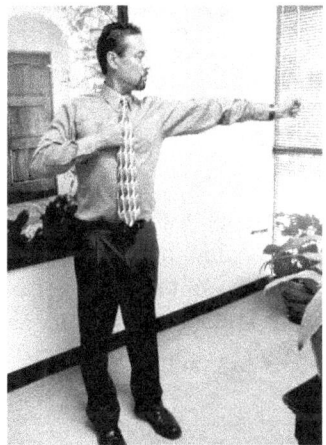

Punch with Eye Glaring

Stand with feet slightly wider than hip distance apart. Making sure that tailbone is tucked under spine, bring hands up so that hands and wrists are in line with elbows, palms facing up, elbows pressed against ribcage. Ball fists and draw elbows back until wrists are pressed against ribcage. Give me your best Kung Fu glare as you punch with right hand, slowly rotating hand so that palm faces ground, moving slowly like you were punching in mud. Pull hand back and repeat with left hand. Repeat 3 to 4 times.

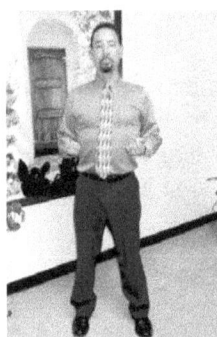 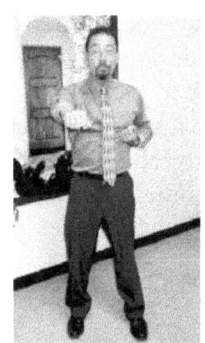

Chair Squats

Begin by sitting on a chair with feet hip distance apart. Knees should be aligned directly over ankles. Sit up tall and bring arms out in front of you at shoulder height with palms of hands pointed in towards the center line of body. Stand, then drop buttocks down as if to sit, trying to keep as much weight *off* chair as you can when coming down to seated position. Press back up to starting position. Repeat 10 times.

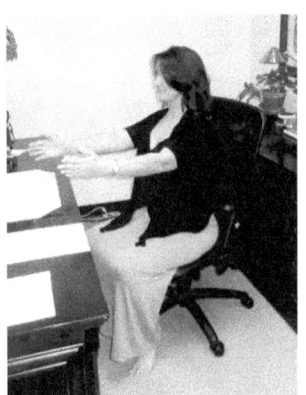 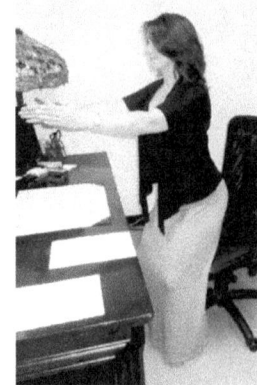

Chair Dips

Sit on an immovable chair or desk. Place hands on either side of hips, with palms flat on desk or seat of chair and fingers pointed forward. With feet on floor, walk feet as far away from you as you can, sliding buttocks off edge of chair or desk. After buttocks have cleared edge of chair or desk and are hovering off ground, body supported by arms and feet, keep knees bent and aligned over the ankles. If you would like a little more of a challenge, extend legs and balance on heels. Keeping core engaged and butt lifted, lower body down towards ground, then press back up to starting position. Repeat for 10 seconds.

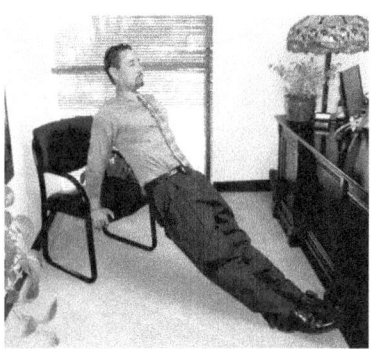 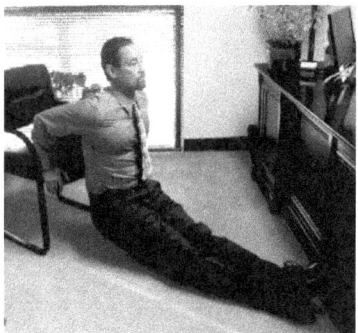

Incline Push-Ups

Stand 3 to 4 feet from a desk or wall. Bring yourself into push-up position with hands on desk or wall and feet on floor. Hands should be directly below shoulders and spine should be long, making sure that hips don't sag or bottom isn't sticking up in the air; body should be angled from ground to desk. From this position, lower chest down to desk, then press back up to starting position. Repeat for 10 seconds.

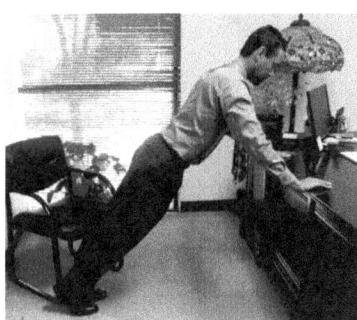 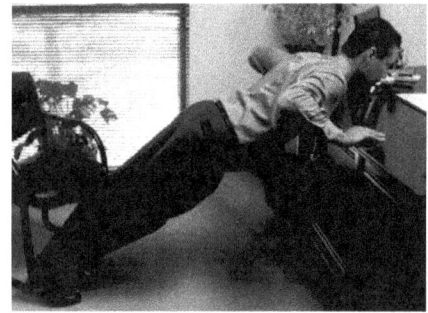

Leg Pull-Downs

Sitting down on an immoveable chair or desk, place hands on either side of hips, palms flat on chair or desk with fingers pointed in front of you. Walk feet as far away from you as you can, sliding buttocks off the edge of chair or desk. After buttocks have cleared edge of chair or desk and are hovering off ground with body weight supported by arms, extend legs and balance on heels. Keeping core engaged and butt lifted, press left heel firmly into ground and lift right foot as high as you can and hold it up. Bring right foot back down, pressing right heel firmly into ground, then lift left foot as high as you can and hold it. Bring left foot down. Repeat on both sides 10 times.

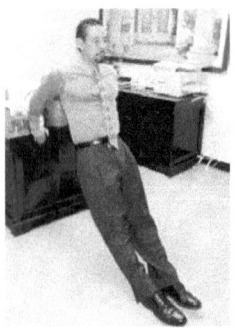 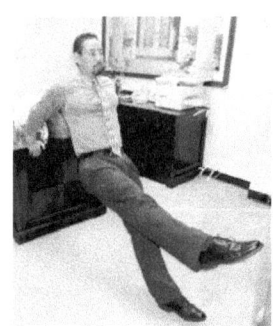

Wide Leg Turnout Squat

Stand with arms folded at chest. Spread legs twice hip distance apart with toes pointed outward at a 45-degree angle from mid-line of body. Bend knees, dropping buttocks down towards floor as if you were going to sit in a chair. Be sure to keep torso as upright as possible. Return to starting position and repeat 10 times.

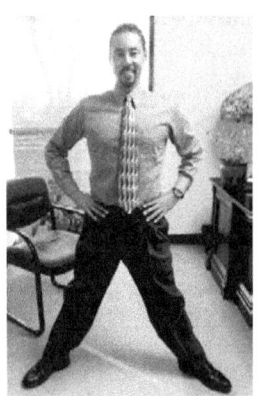 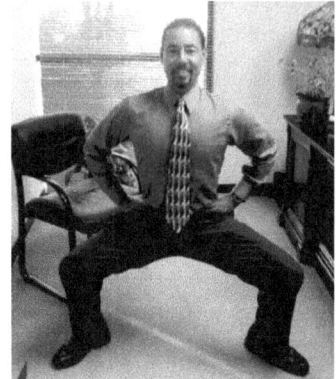

Lunge

Stand with feet slightly wider than hip distance apart. Place both hands on hips. Step forward approximately 18 to 24 inches with right foot. Bend left knee and slowly kneel until left knee touches or almost touches floor. Be sure to keep torso upright and spine long. Keeping feet where they are, slowly stand, then lower left knee back to floor. Repeat 10 times, then switch sides.

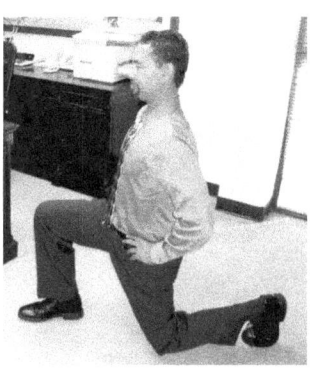 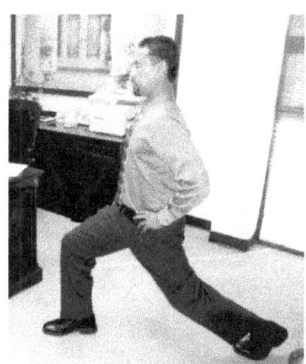

Lateral Raises

Stand with feet slightly wider than hip distance apart and arms down at sides. Keeping arms long and straight, raise them until they reach shoulder height, then lower them back to sides. Repeat 10 times.

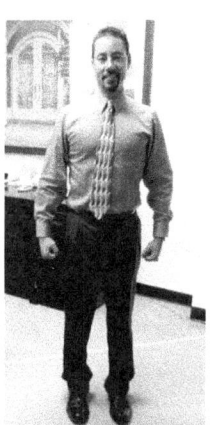 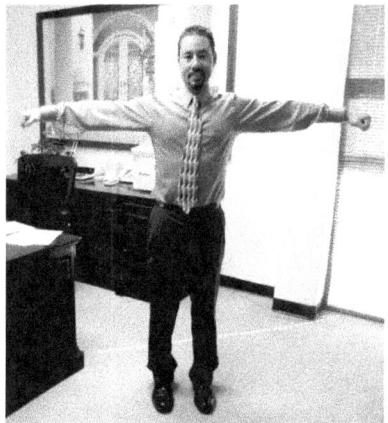

Pushing the Wall

Stand facing a wall that has no furniture in front of it and no pictures that will interfere with you leaning into it. Rest both hands on wall at chest height. Bend elbows slightly. Step back as far as you can with right foot, then press into wall firmly. Continue to press into wall for 10 seconds. Switch legs and repeat.

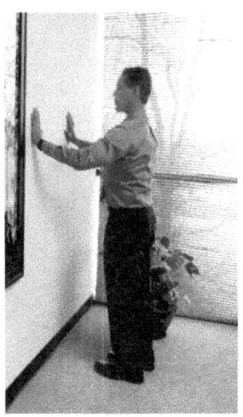 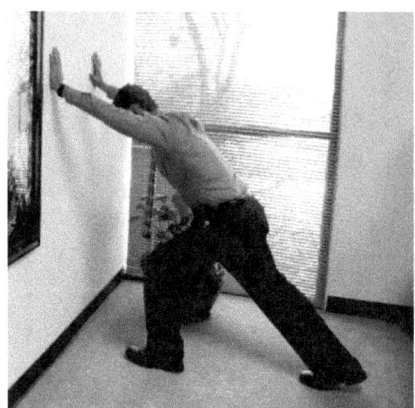

Static Chest Press

This movement can be done either standing or seated. Bring palms of hands together in front of chest. Press hands together as hard as you can and continue to press together for 10 seconds. Take arms down to sides, then swing arms in big circles a few times.

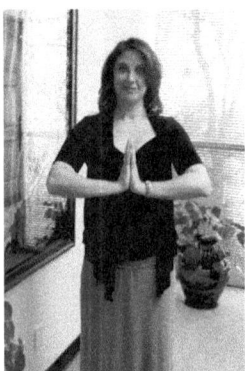

The next 3 movements can be done empty-handed or you can add hand weights, canned goods, full water bottles, etc.

Bicep Curls

Stand with feet slightly wider than hip distance apart. Drop arms down to sides, keeping elbows against rib cage. With palms facing forward, bring hands up to shoulder height then lower down again. Repeat for 1 minute.

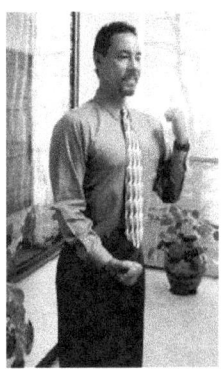
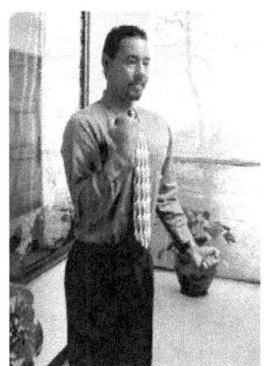

Shoulder Press

Stand with feet slightly wider than hip distance apart. Take arms out to sides and bend elbows. Hands should come to just above shoulders with palms facing upward as if supporting a tray in each hand. Press hands up until arms are completely extended, then lower back down to complete shoulder press. Repeat for 1 minute.

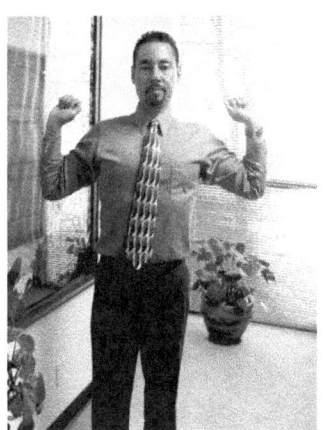
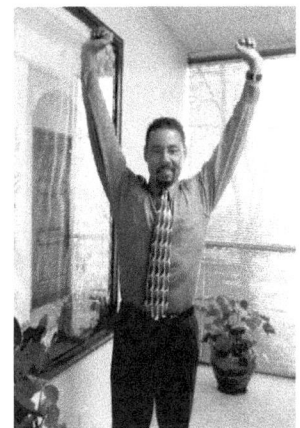

Now that you've perused the movements, you might be thinking "Kent, this is crazy! I almost killed myself doing 30 minutes of P90X every day for two weeks and didn't lose a pound, so how are *these* moves going to help me lose weight?!" My response to you is (in my best Zen master voice): be patient, grasshopper, and all will be revealed.

Let's start simple. Do you know what the difference is in terms of number of calories burned per hour between sitting absolutely still and standing absolutely still? Sixty calories, that's the difference. For the average American, standing absolutely still will burn 60 more calories over the course of an hour than if sitting absolutely still. Ok, so maybe that doesn't sound like that many calories. I mean, heck, that's not even a quarter of a snickers bar.

But when you add up the time we spend commuting to work, sitting at our desks, and parked in front of the TV or surfing social media at night, most of us sit for between 7 and 11 hours a day. And that, my friends, comes out to between 420-660 calories *every day*. You would have to walk at a pace of three miles per hour for two hours (in other words, six miles) to burn even the low end of those numbers. Now keep in mind, these numbers are just for standing absolutely still. Think about how many calories you would burn if you started balancing, walking around, swinging your arms, and stretching. These simple movements are meant to get you used to getting up and moving around on a regular basis, with the added benefits of improving your balance, strengthening your muscles, improving flexibility, and oxygenating and energizing your body.

Remember if you're doing the things I describe in chapter 3, you're up and moving around more already-- adding these desk exercises is simply building that "Sydney effect." Keep in mind that exercise has been proven to have a positive *cumulative* effect, which means that in terms of health benefits, 40 minutes is 40 minutes—even if you break it up into little bitty, five-minute pieces. If you were to do these movements for 5 minutes every hour for 8 hours, that adds up to 40 minutes of movement, and all without ever stepping foot in the gym.

Chapter 6

The Upside of Exercise

(Before starting this or any other exercise program you should check with your physician to be sure that the activities are right for you and your current health.)

Exercise sucks! At least that's what most people think. I don't happen to be one of them, but I do understand why some people might not like doing the thing that I have embraced for most of my life. It's hard work, it's time consuming, it can be downright painful, and it forces us to do things that simply don't come naturally to many of us. There are some really good reasons to do exercise, though, and most of them have to do with your overall health. For example, regular exercise can improve bone health, creating stronger healthier bones and lowering your risk of osteoporosis; it can improve lung function and increase lung capacity, improving oxygenation to all the cells of the body; it can improve muscle tone and muscle strength; and it can help lower stress levels by increasing "soothing" brain chemicals like serotonin, dopamine, and norepinephrine.

What's really amazing, though, is that, according to a 2010 study from the University of California, San Francisco, exercise may actually work on a cellular level to reverse the toll of stress on our aging process. Researchers found that stressed-out women who exercised vigorously for an average of 45 minutes over a three day period had cells that showed fewer signs of aging compared to women who were stressed and inactive. Working out also helps us to mentally let go of things that are troubling us "by altering blood flow to those areas in the brain involved in triggering us to relive these stressful thoughts again and again," says study coauthor Elissa Epel, an associate professor of psychiatry at UCSF. It also has some other surprising benefits for brain health. Research suggests that by doing high intensity exercise (burning at least 350 calories) at least 3 times a week, you can reduce symptoms of depression as effectively as antidepressants.

Exercise can also improve your ability to learn. Exercise increases the level of brain chemicals called "growth factors" which help make new brain cells and establish new connections between brain cells to help us learn. Complicated activities, like playing tennis or taking a dance class, provide the biggest brain boost. You're challenging your brain even more when you have to think about coordination, explains one researcher.

According to the Alzheimer's Research Center, exercise is one of the best weapons against the disease. Exercise appears to protect the hippocampus, which governs memory and spatial navigation, and is one of the first brain regions to succumb to Alzheimer's-related damage. A recent study published in the *Archives of Neurology* suggests that a daily walk or jog could lower the risk of Alzheimer's—or at the very least dull its impact once it has begun. In 2000, Dutch researchers found that inactive men who were genetically prone to Alzheimer's were four times more likely to develop the disease than those who carried the trait but worked out regularly.

In terms of weight loss, we've already talked about the direct calorie burn from exercise, but there is also a secondary benefit. Certain forms of exercise affect the metabolism long after you stop doing the actual exercise. For example, you burn calories both during and after strength training because, once you've finished exercising, your body continues to burn calories making and maintaining the muscle tissue. Strength training can actually boost your metabolism by 15%, which can be a huge help in any weight loss strategy.

Another type of exercise that can help rev up your metabolism and burn fat is interval training. Interval training is simply walking, jogging, biking, or swimming at a high intensity pace for a specific amount of time or distance, then slowing down to a moderate pace for a specific amount of time or distance. Why is this form of training so good for weight loss? It's a double-whammy. It burns more fat than traditional aerobic training in a shorter period of time and it forces your body to work at a higher metabolic rate after the workout is over. Why? At rest, your body needs oxygen and calories from carbohydrates, fat, and protein to maintain life. You need more calories and oxygen to perform exercise, especially at high intensities. Once you stop exercising, your body still requires calories and oxygen as it works to bring you back to resting levels, but your body uses more calories and oxygen after high-intensity interval training than after steady-state aerobic exercise. So with this in mind, our exercise program is going to include these two forms of exercise.

Whoa there tiger, before you pull out the mannequin, dress it in Lululemon and Nike gear and burn me in effigy, let me explain. The workout program I've created for you is short, (less than 20 minutes) simple, and requires just a couple of pieces equipment that are inexpensive and easy to find. By incorporating this program into your day you will notice the fat start to melt away and you will literally see your body begin to change shape as you tone and sculpt your muscles.

I have put together a four week program for you that starts at a beginner level and slowly progresses week by week. You will need to purchase or borrow a set of hand weights. I suggest between 1 and 10 pounds. I don't suggest much more weight than this, even if you currently lift weights, as this program will focus on lifting the weights over a specific time period and not a certain number of repetitions. Getting a set with varying weights will allow you to increase the weight as you get stronger. You can get these weights at almost any sporting goods store or from various online retailers.

http://astore.amazon.com/kenbur-20

You will also need a set of exercise bands that have an attachment that allows you to anchor the bands into a doorway. Again, buying a set will allow you to increase the resistance as your fitness level progresses. These can be purchased at almost any sporting goods store or various online retailers.

http://astore.amazon.com/kenbur-20

Finally, you will need an exercise or stability ball like the one pictured in Chapter 4.

For maximum results I suggest you do the strength training three times a week and the interval training three times a week, which simply means you will be fitting in 15-20 minutes of exercise six days a week. For less than maximum results you can shave a couple of days off that number.

Now, because I'm so confident in the research in sedentary studies and the conclusions that the doctors and scientists have come to in regards to everyday activity and weight loss, I'm going to say something I never thought I would say…in fact, I'm not sure I can say it…(*Gulp*) The exercise portion of this program is *optional.* Did you hear that? It sounded like my exercise physiology professor just rolled over in his grave, or maybe that was the sound of the Royal and Ancient Society of Celebrity Trainers changing the secret handshake to exclude me from future meetings. Oh well.

The Exercise Program

(This program was designed to be done either

in your home or in a gym)

Week 1

Strength training

You should do this program 3 days this week, allowing a day in between workouts (i.e. Monday, Wednesday, and Friday). Do each exercise and then move on to the next exercise without resting in between.

Incline pushups

Get on hands and knees in front of a step or bench. Bring yourself into push-up position with hands on step or bench and feet or knees on floor. Hands should be directly below shoulders and spine should be long, making sure that hips don't sag or bottom isn't sticking up in the air; body should be angled from ground to step. From this position, lower chest down to step then press back up to starting position. Repeat for 50 seconds.

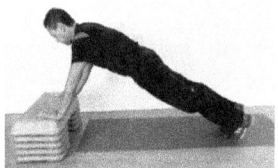 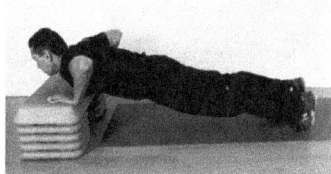

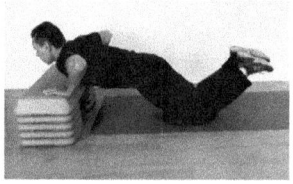

Modification

Chair dips

Sit on an immovable chair or desk. Place hands on either side of hips, with palms flat on desk or seat of chair and fingers pointed forward. With feet on floor, walk feet as far away from you as you can, sliding buttocks off edge of chair or desk. After buttocks have cleared edge of chair or desk and are hovering off ground, body supported by arms and feet, keep knees bent and aligned over ankles. For more of a challenge, extend legs and balance on heels. Keeping core engaged and butt lifted, lower body down towards ground, then press back up to starting position. Repeat for 50 seconds.

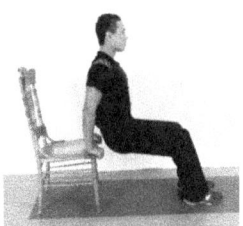 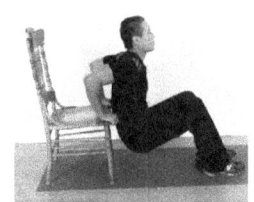

Bicep Curls

Stand with feet slightly wider than hip distance apart. Holding a 1 to 10 pound dumbbell in each hand, drop arms down to sides, keeping elbows against rib cage. With palms facing forward, bring hands up to shoulder height then lower down again. Repeat for 50 seconds.

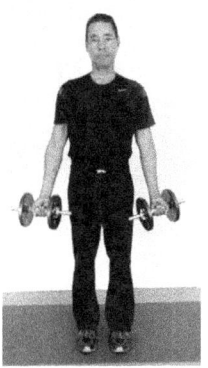 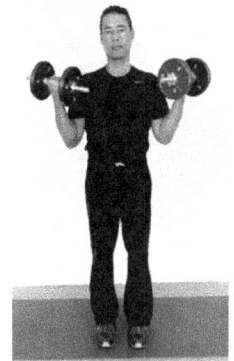

Shoulder Press

Stand with feet slightly wider than hip distance apart. Holding a 1 to 10 pound dumbbell in each hand, take arms out to sides and bend elbows. Hands should come to just above shoulders and palms should be facing upward as if supporting a tray in each hand. Press hands up until arms are completely extended, then lower back down to complete the shoulder press. Repeat for 50 seconds.

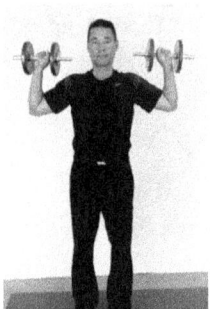 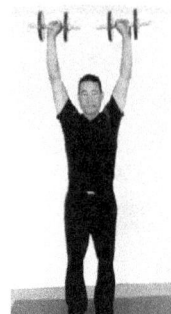

Squat

Holding a 1 to 10 pound weight in each hand, bring feet a little wider than hip distance apart. Keeping back straight and leaning forward as little as possible, slowly lower bottom down as if you were going to sit in a chair. Go as low as you comfortably can, then bring yourself back up to starting position. Repeat for 50 seconds.

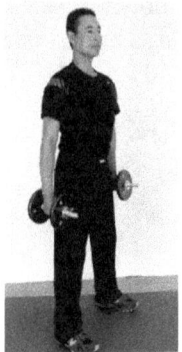 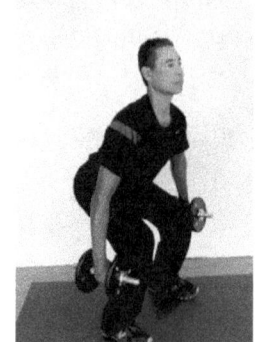

Lunge

Stand with feet slightly wider than hip distance apart. Holding a 1 to 10 pound dumbbell in each hand, step forward approximately 18 to 24 inches with right foot. Bend left knee and slowly kneel until left knee touches or almost touches floor. Be sure to keep torso upright and spine long. Keeping feet where they are, slowly stand, then switch sides. Repeat, alternating sides for 50 seconds.

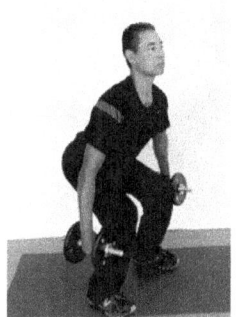 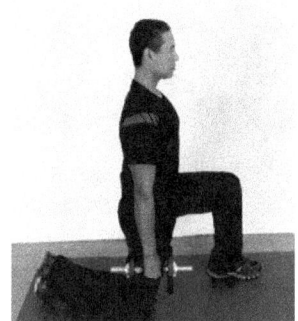

Crunches

Lie on back with knees bent and feet flat on floor, hip-width apart. Place hands behind head so thumbs are behind ears. Hold elbows out to sides but rounded slightly in. Tilt chin slightly, leaving a few inches of space between chin and chest. Gently pull abdominals inward. Curl up and forward so that head, neck, and shoulder blades lift off floor. Hold for a moment at the top of the movement and then lower slowly back down. Continue for 50 seconds.

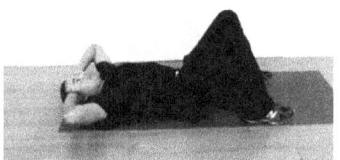 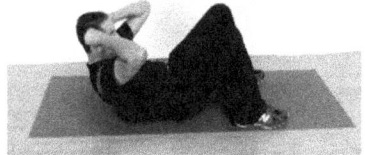

Plank

Begin on elbows, forearms and knees, then draw one knee off floor followed by other knee. This brings you into a classic push up position. Keep back flat (don't allow butt to sag or poke up into the air) and hold this position for 50 seconds.

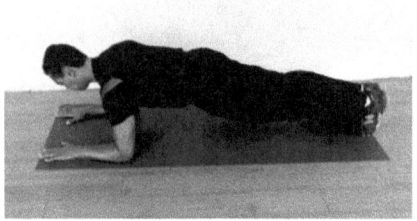

Start from the beginning and go through each exercise once more. This entire workout should take you no more than 16 minutes.

Interval training

You should do this workout 3 days a week on days that you do not strength train. Each exercise has been given an intensity rating based on a perceived exertion test or (PE). This test uses a scale of 1 to 10 to rank how hard it feels like you are working during a given exercise. A ranking of 1 is: I'm almost asleep. A 10 is: Dear lord I'm going to die! A ranking of 1-3 is easy, 4-6 is moderate, and 7-10 is hard. You can do these intervals outside in your neighborhood or on a treadmill walking, jogging, or a combination of the two. They can also be done on a stationary bike or even swimming. For this workout you will need a timer or a stop watch that you can easily carry with you.

Minutes 1-3

Begin at an easy pace (PE 2-3) for 3 minutes to warm up your body.

Minute 4-5

Pick up your pace to moderate (PE 4-5) for 1 minute

Minutes 5-6

Pick up the pace to fast (PE 7-8) for 1 minute

Minutes 6-9

Slow down to a moderate pace (PE 4-5) for 3 minutes

Minutes 9-10

Pick up the pace to fast (PE 7-8) for 1 minute

Minutes 10-13

Slow down to a moderate pace (PE 4-5) for 3 minutes

Minutes 13-14

Pick up the pace to fast (PE 7-8) for 1 minute

Minutes 14-17

Slow down to a moderate pace (PE 4-5) for 3 minutes

Minutes 17-20

Slow down to an easy pace (PE 2-3) cool down

Week 2

Strength training

You should do this program 3 days this week allowing a day in between workouts (i.e. Monday, Wednesday, and Friday). Do each exercise and then move on to the next exercise without resting in between.

Push up

Begin on hands and knees, then draw one knee off floor, followed by other knee. his brings you into a classic push up position. Keep back flat (don't allow butt to sag or poke up into the air). Lower chest down to floor then push back up to starting position. Repeat for 50 seconds (if you need to stop and rest that's ok, just start again as soon as you feel you can).

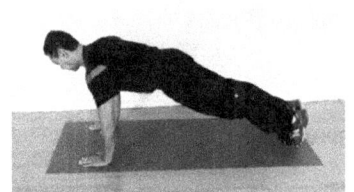 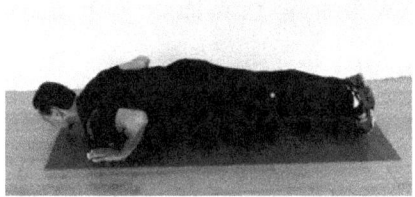

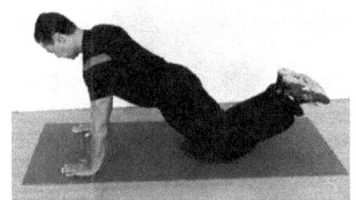 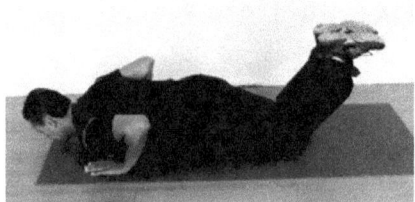

Modification

Triceps extension

Stand with feet slightly wider than hip distance apart. Take a 1 to10 pound dumbbell in both hands and lift it up overhead (weight should be directly over crown of head). Bend elbows and lower weight down behind head, then lift it back overhead. Repeat for 50 seconds.

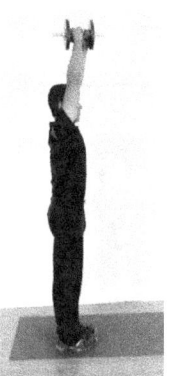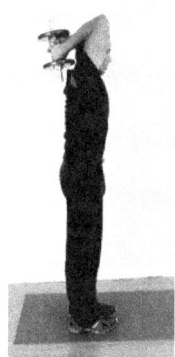

Hammer curls

Stand with feet slightly wider than hip distance apart. Holding a 1 to 10 pound dumbbell in each hand, drop arms down to sides, with palms of hands turned inward. Keeping elbows against rib cage, bring hands up to shoulder height, then lower down again. Repeat for 50 seconds.

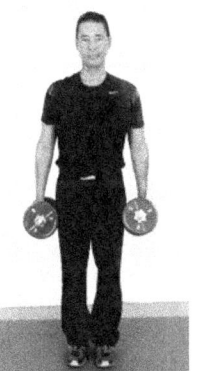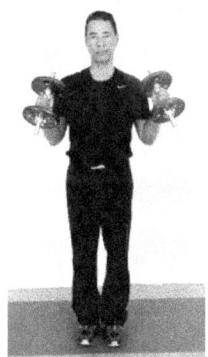

Lateral Raises

Stand with feet slightly wider than hip distance apart. Holding a 1 to 10 pound dumbbell in each hand, drop arms down to sides. Keeping arms bent, raise elbows and hands up until they reach shoulder height, then lower back to your sides. Repeat for 50 seconds.

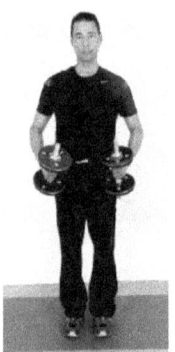 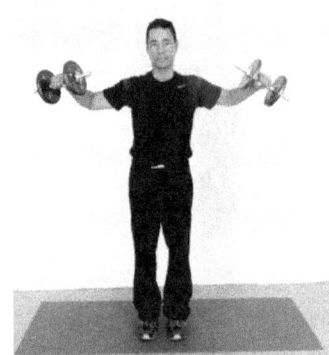

Wide Leg Squat

Stand holding a 1 to 10 pound dumbbell in each hand. Spread legs twice hip distance apart with toes pointed outward at a 45-degree angle from mid-line of body. Bend knees as you drop buttocks down towards floor as if you were going to sit in a chair, being sure to keep torso as upright as possible. Return to starting position. Repeat for 50 seconds.

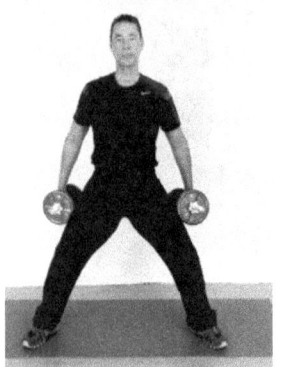 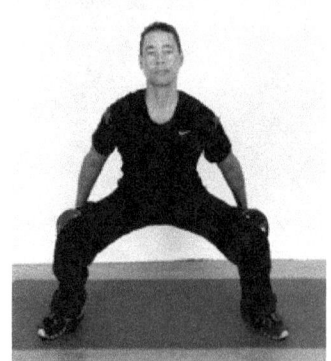

Lunge

Stand with feet slightly wider than hip distance apart. Holding a 1 to 10 pound dumbbell in each hand, step forward approximately 18 to 24 inches with right foot. Bend left knee and slowly kneel until left knee touches or almost touches floor. Be sure to keep torso upright and spine long. Keeping feet where they are, slowly stand, then switch sides. Repeat, alternating sides for 50 seconds.

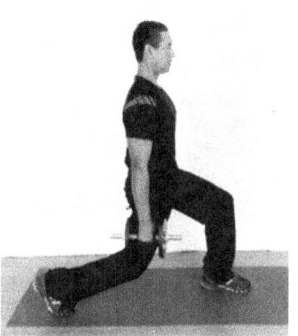 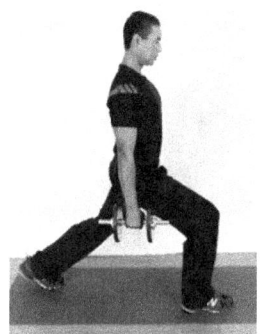

Bicycle Crunch

Lie flat on floor with lower back pressed to ground and contract core muscles. With hands gently holding head, lift knees to about a 45-degree angle. Slowly, at first, go through a bicycle pedal motion, alternately touching elbows to opposite knees as you twist back and forth. Breathe evenly throughout the exercise. Continue for 50 seconds.

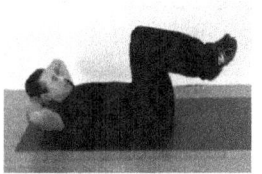 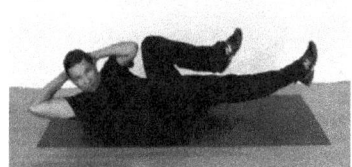

Modified Alternate Arm/Leg Plank

Get down hands and knees (hands directly beneath shoulders and knees directly beneath hips). Keeping torso absolutely still, raise right hand off floor and reach forward, keeping right elbow and wrist in line with shoulder. At the same time lift left knee off floor, extending left leg back and away from body and keeping ankle and knee in line with hip. Hold for a count of 5 then come back to starting position. Repeat with opposite arm and leg. Repeat, switching back and forth for 50 seconds.

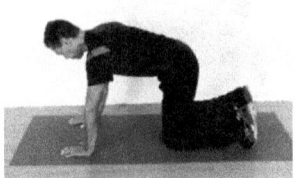 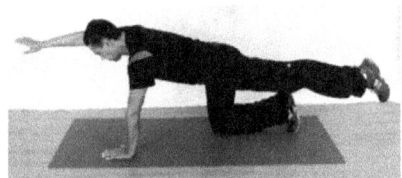

Start from the beginning and go through each exercise one more time. This entire workout should take you no more than 16 minutes.

Interval training

You should do this workout 3 days a week on days that you do not strength train. Each exercise has been given an intensity rating based on a perceived exertion test or (PE). This test uses a scale of 1 to 10 to rank how hard it feels like you are working during a given exercise. A ranking of 1 is: I'm almost asleep. A 10 is: Dear lord I'm going to die! A ranking of 1-3 is easy, 4-6 is moderate, and 7-10 is hard. You can do these intervals outside in your neighborhood or on a treadmill walking, jogging, or a combination of the two. They can also be done on a stationary bike or even swimming. For this workout you will need a timer or a stop watch that you can easily carry with you.

Minutes 1-3

Begin at an easy pace (PE 2-3) for 3 minutes to warm up your body.

Minute 4-5

Pick up your pace to moderate (PE 4-5) for 1 minute

Minutes 5-6

Pick up the pace to fast (PE 7-8) for 1 minute

Minutes 6-9

Slow down to a moderate pace (PE 4-5) for 3 minutes

Minutes 9-10

Pick up the pace to fast (PE 7-8) for 1 minute

Minutes 10-13

Slow down to a moderate pace (PE 4-5) for 3 minutes

Minutes 13-14

Pick up the pace to fast (PE 7-8) for 1 minute

Minutes 14-17

Slow down to a moderate pace (PE 4-5) for 3 minutes

Minutes 17-20

Slow down to an easy pace (PE 2-3) cool down

Week 3

Strength training

Chest Press with Resistance Bands

Anchor resistance band in a door or wrap it around a pole, tree, bedpost or other stationary object. Make sure resistance band will be lined up with middle of chest (i.e., band should run under arms). Stand in front of resistance band and grab both handles with an overhand grip. Walk away from object holding band until desired resistance is reached. Keep chest up, back straight and feet positioned with one foot in front of the other. Knees should have a slight bend. Having wrists aligned with elbows (straight forearm), press handles forward and bring them together at top of movement. Squeeze chest and hold for a count of 1. Lower handles back toward starting position in a slow and controlled manner, feeling stretch of pectoral muscles. Repeat for 50 seconds.

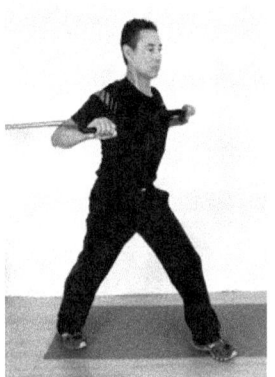 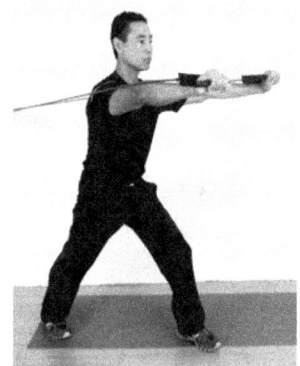

Triceps Extensions with Resistance Bands

Secure resistance band to bottom of door and, facing away from door, grab both handles with palms facing up towards ceiling (bands should be behind you). Bring hands above head, palms facing forward and elbows bent at forehead level. Press hands upward until elbows are straight, then return hands to starting position. Repeat for 50 seconds.

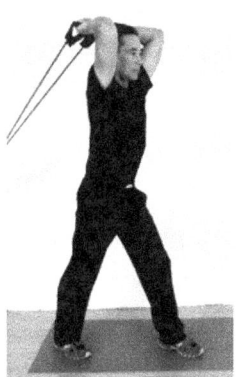 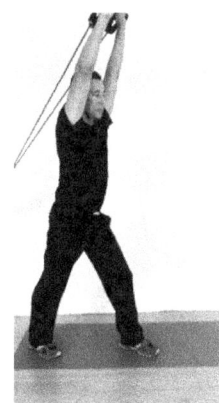

Biceps Curls with Resistance Bands

Grasp ends of resistance band and hold hands facing chest. Stand with feet hip width apart, and place center of band under one foot as an anchor. Keep wrists straight while holding hand bars. Don't bend wrists toward you or away from you. Maintain a slow, deliberate movement as you perform a bicep curl exercise with resistance band. Raise forearms toward you, and bend elbows to point where hands stop in front of shoulders. Hold hand bars at shoulder level for a second before releasing arms down. Release arms down, keeping hands facing chest. Keep resistance band taut as you release hands to hip level. Maximum results will come from constant resistance of band during entire movement. Repeat for 50 seconds.

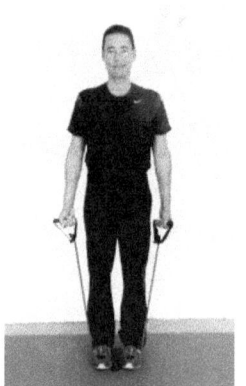 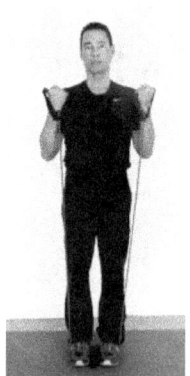

Shoulder Press with Tubing

Place both feet on tube and grasp handles, bringing hands up just over shoulders with elbows bent and palms facing forward. Press arms up over head and then lower. Repeat for 50 seconds.

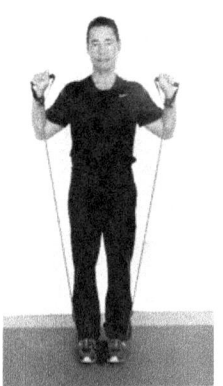 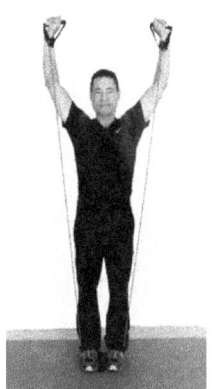

Wall Sit with Ball

Stand facing away from a clear wall surface with an exercise ball behind you. Press ball firmly into wall. Slide down until knees are at about 90-degree angles (or an angle that is comfortable for you) and hold, keeping abs contracted. Hold for 50 seconds.

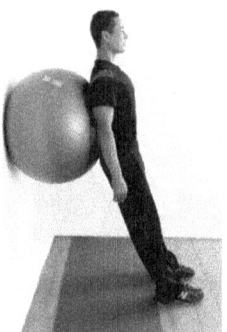 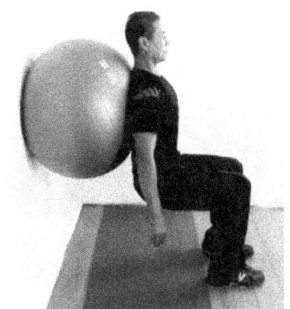

Step Up

Stand facing a secure chair or bench. Step up onto chair or bench with right foot, keeping back tall and head facing forward. Bring both feet up onto chair or bench surface, then step down. Repeat on the other side. Continue to step up and down, alternating feet for 50 seconds.

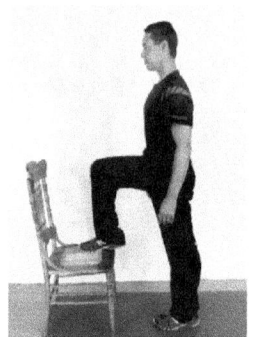 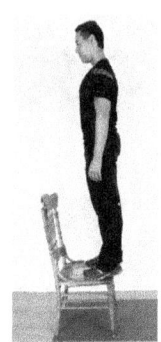

V Sits

Starting in a seated position, contract abdominal muscles and core, and lift legs up to a 45-degree angle. Reach arms straight forward or reach up toward shins as you are able. Maintain good core posture and a strong spine. Hold this "V" position for 50 seconds.

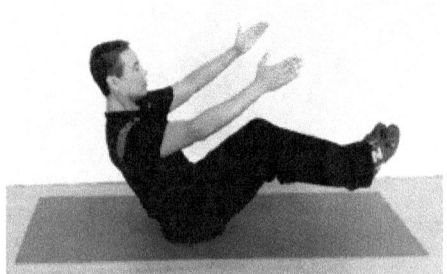

Full Plank

Beginning on elbows, forearms and knees, draw one knee off floor followed by other knee, then bring yourself up to hands. This brings you into a classic push up position. Keep back flat (don't allow butt to sag or poke up into the air) and hold this position for 50 seconds.

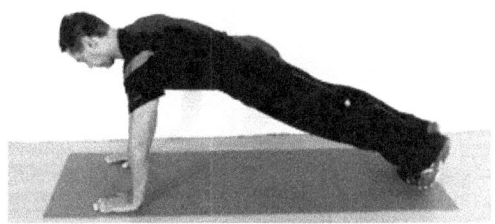

Interval training

You should do this workout 3 days a week on days that you do not strength train. Each exercise has been given an intensity rating based on a perceived exertion test or (PE). This test uses a scale of 1 to 10 to rank how hard it feels like you are working during a given exercise. A ranking of 1is: I'm almost asleep. A 10 is: Dear lord I'm going to die! A ranking of 1-3 is easy, 4-6 is moderate, and 7-10 is hard. You can do these intervals outside in your neighborhood or on a treadmill walking, jogging, or a combination of the two. They can also be done on a stationary bike or even swimming. For this workout you will need a timer or a stop watch that you can easily carry with you.

Minutes 1-3

Begin at an easy pace (PE 2-3) for 3 minutes to warm up your body.

Minute 3-5

Pick up your pace to moderate (PE 4-5) for 2 minutes

Minutes 5-7

Pick up the pace to fast (PE 7-8) for 2 minutes

Minutes 7-10

Slow down to a moderate pace (PE 4-5) for 3 minutes

Minutes 10-12

Pick up the pace to fast (PE 7-8) for 2 minutes

Minutes 12-15

Slow down to a moderate pace (PE 4-5) for 3 minutes

Minutes 15-17

Pick up the pace to fast (PE 7-8) for 2 minutes

Minutes 17-20

Slow down to a moderate pace (PE 4-5) for 3 minutes cool down

Week 4

Chest Fly with Resistance Bands

Anchor band in a doorway or other stationary waist-high fixture and stand with back to band. Holding a handle in each hand, allow band to pull arms slightly behind you. Take a firm stance with one leg behind body for stability. Bring hands together in front of you, insides of fists almost touching. As you move, focus on chest muscles tensing as you bring hands together. Use a slow, controlled motion to get the most out of this exercise. Extend arms out to sides, roughly parallel with floor. Return to starting position, then repeat for 50 seconds.

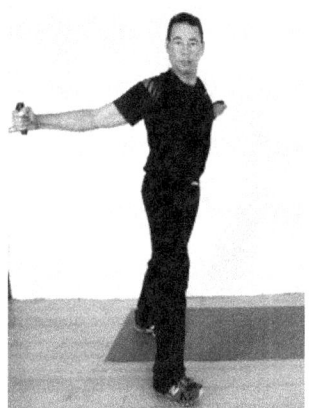 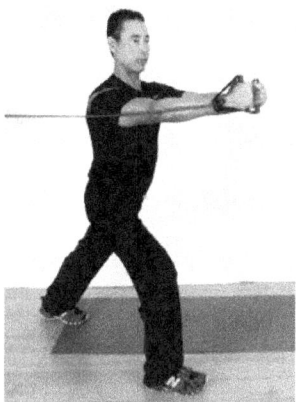

Triceps Pull Downs with Resistance Bands

Anchor resistance band at top of a door, making sure it is above head). Stand in front of resistance band and grab both handles with an overhand grip, then turn away from where resistance band is anchored and walk away from object holding band until desired resistance is reached. Bring hands above head, palms facing forward, elbows bent at forehead level. Press hands forward until elbows are straight then return hands to starting position. Repeat for 50 seconds.

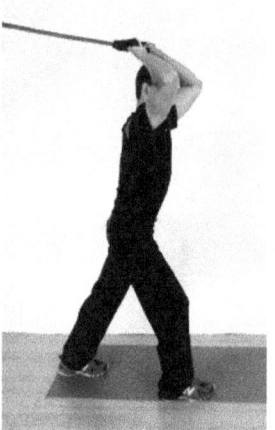 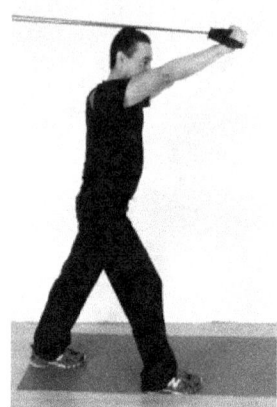

Bicep Wing Curls with Resistance Bands

Grasp ends of resistance band. Stand with feet hip width apart and place center of band itself under one foot as an anchor. Keep wrists straight while holding hand bars. Don't bend wrists toward you or away from you. Rotate both arms outward then maintain a slow, deliberate movement as you pull both hands up towards shoulders. Hold hand bars at shoulder level for 1 second before releasing arms down. Release arms down, keeping hands facing outward. Keep resistance band taut as you release hands to hip level. Maximum results will come from constant resistance of band during entire movement. Repeat for 50 seconds.

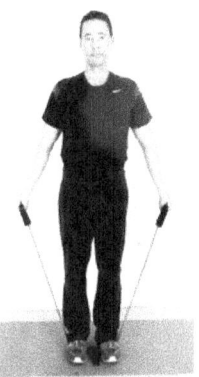 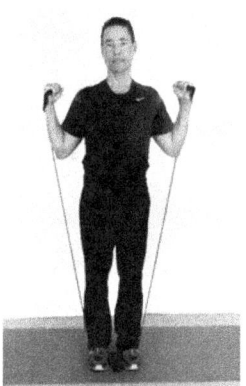

Lateral Raises with Resistance Bands

Grasp ends of resistance band. Stand with feet hip width apart and place center of band under one foot as an anchor. Holding handles of resistance bands in each hand, drop arms down to sides. Keeping arms bent, raise elbows and hands up until they reach shoulder height, then lower them back to sides. Repeat for 50 seconds.

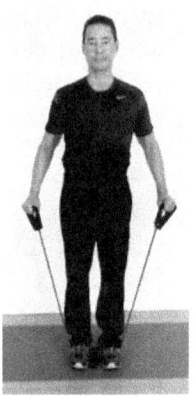 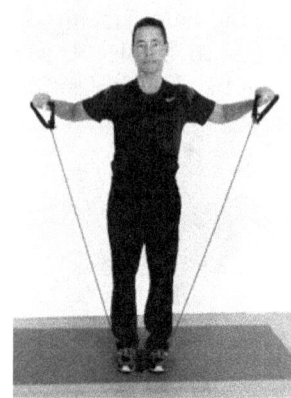

Wide Leg Seated Squat

Stand holding 1 to 10 pound weights in both hands with a stable chair behind you. Spread legs so they are twice hip distance apart with toes pointed outward at a 45-degree angle from mid-line of body. Bend knees and drop buttocks down to chair behind you, keeping torso as upright as possible. Return to starting position. Repeat for 50 seconds.

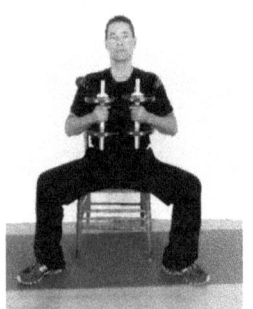 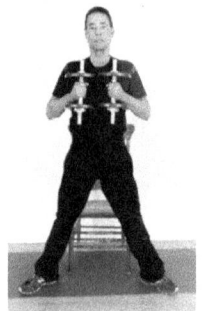

One Legged Lunge

Begin standing with back to a bench or step. Place one leg up on bench or step so that shoelaces are resting on bench. Align front foot forward so you are in a lunging position. Keeping hips rolled under, lunge straight down until back knee is close to ground and front leg is at a 90-degree angle. Pressing through front heel, push up and return to starting position. Do on one side for 25 seconds, then switch to opposite side for 25 seconds.

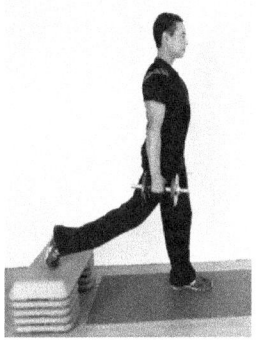 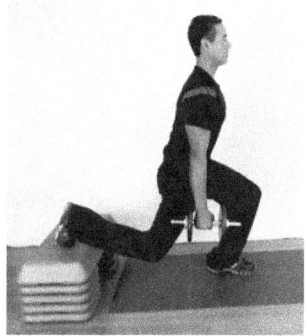

Roll Up

Lie back with legs straight and arms extended above head next to ears. Bring arms forward, tilt chin down, and slowly curl upper body up, reaching hands up towards ceiling. Extend spine upwards, bringing torso up and tall. Slowly lower torso back down to floor one vertebrae at a time, bringing yourself back to starting position. Repeat for 50 seconds.

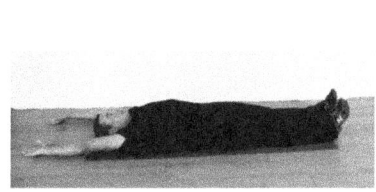 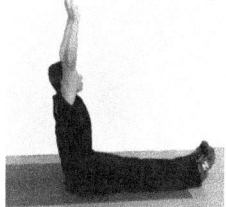

Ball Plank

Put exercise ball on floor under upper body. Lay down on exercise ball face down, keeping it under chest with feet extended away from you, hands gently holding side of ball. Keep torso as still as possible with toes on floor in plank position. Hold position for 50 seconds, keeping ball as still as possible.

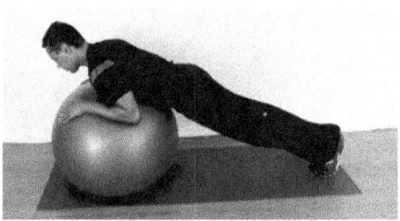

Interval training

You should do this workout 3 days a week on days that you do not strength train. Each exercise has been given an intensity rating based on a perceived exertion test or (PE). This test uses a scale of 1 to 10 to rank how hard it feels like you are working during a given exercise. A ranking of 1 is: I'm almost asleep. A 10 is: Dear lord I'm going to die! A ranking of 1-3 is easy, 4-6 is moderate, and 7-10 is hard. You can do these intervals outside in your neighborhood or on a treadmill walking, jogging, or a combination of the two. They can also be done on a stationary bike or even swimming. For this workout you will need a timer or a stop watch that you can easily carry with you.

Minutes 1-3

Begin at an easy pace (PE 2-3) for 3 minutes to warm up your body.

Minute 3-5

Pick up your pace to moderate (PE 4-5) for 2 minutes

Minutes 5-7

Pick up the pace to fast (PE 7-8) for 2 minutes

Minutes 7-10

Slow down to a moderate pace (PE 4-5) for 3 minutes

Minutes 10-12

Pick up the pace to fast (PE 7-8) for 2 minutes

Minutes 12-15

Slow down to a moderate pace (PE 4-5) for 3 minutes

Minutes 15-17

Pick up the pace to fast (PE 7-8) for 2 minutes

Minutes 17-20

Slow down to a moderate pace (PE 4-5) for 3 minutes cool down

When you have finished this four week program you can continue doing the final weeks' exercises, slowly increasing the weight and intensity. You can also visit my website, www.kentburden.com, where I have 15-20 minute exercise programs on DVD available for purchase

Of course there are many other programs out there as well; the main thing is finding a program that is right for you. The best exercise program in the world is simply the one *YOU WILL DO* on a regular basis.

Exercise Sucks!

Chapter 7

Controlling Stress for Weight Loss

Let's face it, between work, family, and the pressures of living our hectic modern lives we live in a very stressful world. Stress is a part of everyone's day-to day life. But did you know that stress can cause you to gain weight and may even be why you can't seem to lose weight? It's true. Stress affects us physically and mentally in a variety of ways. From the physical side of things, prolonged stress can cause a cascade of hormones in the body, including one called cortisol which is a key player in the body's fight or flight response. Cortisol is vital for proper physical functioning, so it is actually healthy in small doses. However, when the body perceives a threat, whether real or imagined, and that threat seems to be imminent, the fight or flight response is activated. During this reaction, cortisol release increases to allow for a burst of energy and other physical changes that help us get the hell out of dodge or turn and kick some butt. After the threat is gone the body undergoes the relaxation response and all systems return to normal.

However, when the stress sticks around (chronic stress), homeostasis is never reached and the body maintains increased levels of cortisol, which can be damaging to the body in many ways. One side effect of increased cortisol in the body can be weight gain, especially in the abdominal area, which can lead to more negative health consequences than fat stored in other areas of the body. Cortisol has been shown to slow metabolism, which is why stress can make you gain weight and make it more difficult to lose weight. People who are constantly stressed also tend to crave fatty, sugary, and salty foods, none of which are very good for the old waistline.

On the emotional side, when stressed we tend to eat whether we're hungry or not, noshing away on just about anything edible in the general vicinity. On top of that chronic stress tends to leave us feeling physically and emotionally drained. This can lead us to the drive thru window for dinner because we don't feel like we have the energy to cook. All it takes is one look at the calorie counts on fast food menus to figure out how that's going to affect the number on the bathroom scale. Add these hormonal and emotional weight gain contributors to sitting around the office and house all day, and you end up with the perfect combination for expanded waistlines and bulging booties.

So what can you do about your stress levels (besides going postal or selling everything you own and running off to Bora Bora to sell handmade jewelry on the beach)?

Here are a few recommendations regarding stress from Doctor Edward T. Creagan, M.D. of the Mayo Clinic:

-Recognize the warning signs of stress, such as anxiety, irritability and muscle tension.

-Before eating, ask yourself why you're eating — are you truly hungry or do you feel stressed or anxious?

-If you're tempted to eat when you're not hungry, find a distraction.

-Don't skip meals, especially breakfast.

-Identify comfort foods and keep them out of your home or office.

-Keep a record of your behavior and eating habits so that you can look for patterns and connections — and then figure out how to overcome them.

-Learn problem-solving skills so that you can anticipate challenges and cope with setbacks.

-Practice relaxation skills, such as yoga, massage, or meditation.

-Engage in regular physical activity or exercise.

-Get adequate sleep.

-Get encouragement from supportive friends and family.

I personally find that doing yoga on a regular basis helps me deal with the stresses that come with everyday life, and when things get really bad I indulge myself with a massage. But the thing I find most affective in dealing with everyday stress is meditation. When most people think of meditation they think of monks hidden away in temple high on a mountain top somewhere but the definition of meditation is actually quite simple: "to contemplate or bring silence to the mind" and there are many different techniques for doing that. To help you get a handle on your stress, I'm going to suggest some simple breathing exercises. These simple meditation breathing techniques can be done almost anywhere (without your coworkers, neighbors, and friends staring at you in disbelief) and are amazingly affective. Each of these techniques can be used for very specific situations but should be practiced on a regular basis to make them as effective as possible.

4-7-8 Breath

This exercise is utterly simple, takes almost no time, requires no equipment and can be done anywhere. Although you can do the exercise in any position, it is best to sit with your back straight while learning the exercise. Place the tip of your tongue against the ridge of tissue just behind your upper front teeth, and keep it there through the entire exercise. You will be exhaling through your mouth around your tongue; try pursing your lips slightly if this seems awkward.

Exhale completely through your mouth, making a whoosh sound.

Close your mouth and inhale quietly through your nose to a mental count of **4**.

Hold your breath for a count of **7**.

Exhale completely through your mouth, making a whoosh sound to a count of **8**.

This is one breath. Repeat the cycle 3 more times for a total of 4 breaths. (From Dr. Andrew Weil's website www.drweil.com)

Cooling breath

This breath is meant to cool the nervous system and mind. This simple breathing technique is a great way to relieve stress and cool down a hot temper.

Stick your tongue out of your mouth and curl it, creating a small straw- like tube with your tongue.

Slowly and smoothly suck air in through your tongue filling your lungs with air. Draw your tongue into your mouth and close your lips.

Hold your breath for a count of 5, then exhale slowly and smoothly through your nostrils.

Repeat 3 times.

Bellows Breath

The Bellows Breath is adapted from a yogic breathing technique. Its aim is to raise vital energy and increase alertness.

> Inhale and exhale rapidly through your nose, keeping your mouth closed but relaxed. Your breaths in and out should be equal in duration, but as short as possible. (This is a noisy breathing exercise.)

> Try for 3 in-and-out breath cycles per second. This produces a quick movement of the diaphragm, suggesting a bellows. Breathe normally after each cycle.

> Do not do for more than 15 seconds on your first try. Each time you practice the Bellows Breath, you can increase your time by 5 seconds or so, until you reach a full minute.

If done properly, you may feel invigorated, comparable to the heightened awareness you feel after a good workout. You should feel the effort at the back of the neck, the diaphragm, the chest and the abdomen. Try this breathing exercise the next time you need an energy boost and feel yourself reaching for a cup of coffee. (From Dr. Andrew Weil's website www.drweil.com)

Alternate Nostril Breathing

Alternate nostril breathing creates optimum function of both sides of the brain, improves mood, strengthens the lungs, and energizes the body.

> Close off the right nostril with your right thumb, then inhale through the left nostril to a three-count,
>
> Hold your breath for an eight-count.
>
> Release your thumb from your right nostril and exhale through the right nostril for a count of 6 as you close off the left nostril with your left thumb.
>
> Now inhale through your right nostril for a three-count and repeat this on both sides for 1 to 3 minutes.

By getting a handle on your stress you put another tool in your tool belt to help you control your weight. The more tools you have the higher the chance for a successful outcome of the project. At least, that's what my 7th grade shop teacher Mr. Williams told me.

Exercise Sucks!

Chapter 8
Conclusion

This book is designed to be a straightforward guide to losing weight while doing a minimal amount of exercise. First I went over how important regular activity is to your health and weight loss goals. Then I, talked about ways you can eat for a healthier, lighter you. Then I showed you how to be more active—bumping up the little everyday activities you used to do without thinking, and supercharging your calorie burn while doing them. From there I introduced tools that can help you keep track of how active you really are and help you be even more active.

Then we upped the ante with keystone habit movements that can start you down the path to being more active by doing simple movements every hour and adding even more activity to your day. I also showed you exercises, that when done for just 15-20 minutes a day could speed your weight loss even more. Finally, I explained how stress can affect your ability to lose weight and gave you techniques to minimize that stress.

And I have really good news. Not only will incorporating these techniques and lifestyle changes help you lose weight, they may actually lengthen your life and lower your risk of developing lifestyle diseases such as diabetes, heart disease, stroke and certain types of cancer.

But some of you will want proof that this actually has science behind it. I get that. If you are one of those people, see below for several books I think you might want to read.

Is Your Chair Killing You?, by Kent Burden

Move a Little, Lose a Lot: Use N.E.A.T.* Science to: Burn 2,100 Calories a Week at the Office, Be Smarter in as Little as 3 Hours, Reduce Fatigue by 65%, Extend Your Lifespan by 4 Years, by James Levine, M.D. & Selene Yeager

Sitting Kills, Moving Heals: How Everyday Movement will Prevent Pain, Illness, and Early Death-And Exercise Alone Won't, by Joan Vernikos, Ph.D.

One Small Step Can Change Your Life: The Kaizen Way, by Robert Maurer

In closing, being more active can only be a good thing in your life. After all, it is exactly what your body was designed to do. It is my hope that reading this book and following its principles will improve your overall life, health, and happiness.

You can get more information and find out how to contact me at www.kentburden.com.

Also by Kent Burden

The Kindle Healthy Living Bestseller:

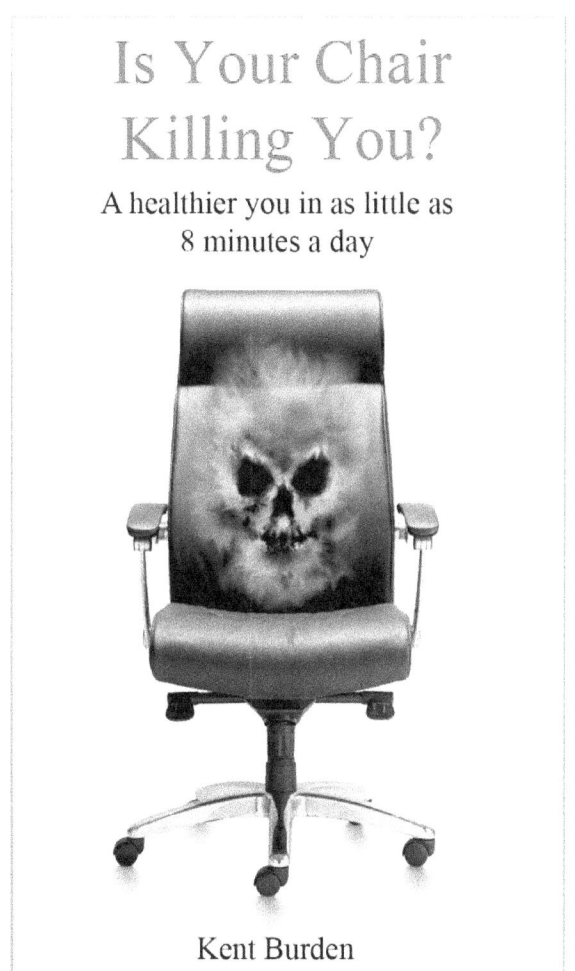

Available on Amazon.com: tinyurl.com/9r74tgp

www.ingramcontent.com/pod-product-compliance
Lightning Source LLC
Chambersburg PA
CBHW072325290526
45794CB00002B/745